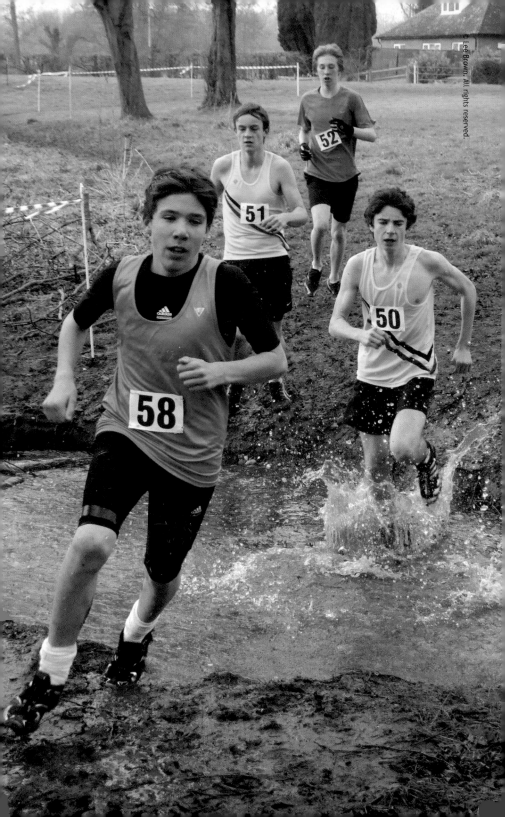

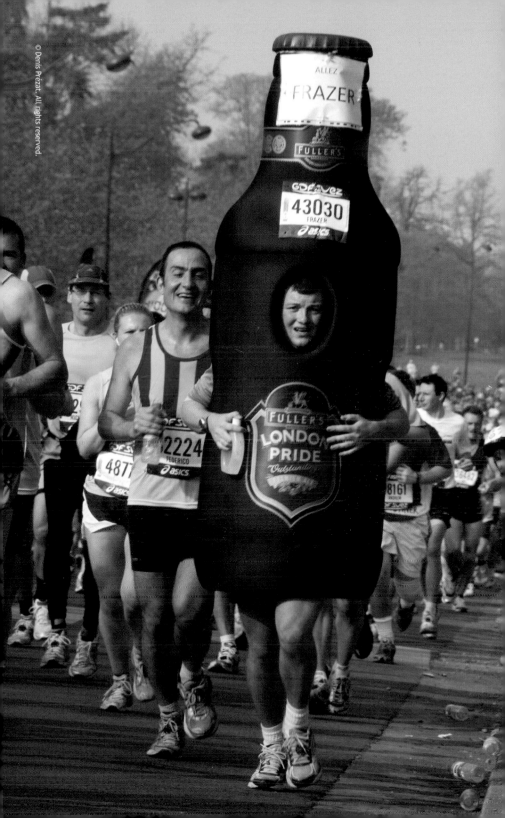

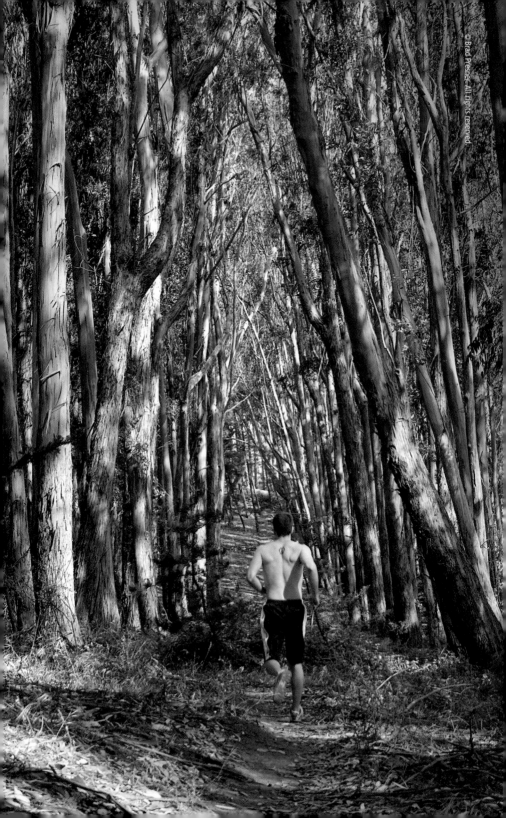

The

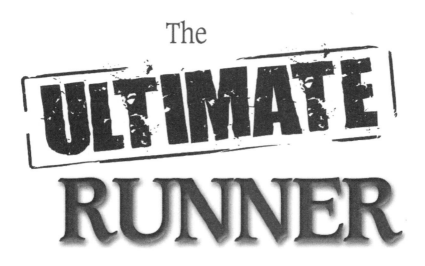

RUNNER

Stories and Advice
to Keep You Moving

Tom Green and Amy Hunold-VanGundy
creators of *Runners' Lounge*

Health Communications, Inc.
HCI Books, the Life Issues Publisher
Deerfield Beach, Florida

www.hcibooks.com
www.ultimatehcibooks.com

We would like to acknowledge the writers and photographers who granted us permission to use their material. Copyright credits for interior photographs appear on each photograph and credits for literary work are listed alphabetically by authors' last names. Contact information as supplied by the photographers and writers can be found in the back matter of this book.

Library of Congress Cataloging-in-Publication Data

Green, Tom.
  The ultimate runner : stories and advice to keep you moving / by Tom Green and Amy J. Hunold-VanGundy.
    p. cm.
  Includes index.
  ISBN-13: 978-0-7573-1439-1
  ISBN-10: 0-7573-1439-2
  1. Running—Miscellanea.   2. Running—Training.   3. Physical fitness.
  I. Hunold-VanGundy, Amy J.   II. Title.
  GV1061.5.G74 2010
  796.42—dc22

                                                            2010006750

©2010 Health Communications, Inc.

Publisher: Health Communications, Inc.
          3201 S.W. 15th Street
          Deerfield Beach, FL 33442-8190

Cover Design: Justin Rotkowitz
Cover Photo: © David De Lossy
Photo Editor: Justin Rotkowitz
Interior Design: Lawna Patterson Oldfield
Interior Formatting: Dawn Von Strolley Grove

To our spouses, children, and family members.
Thank you for the endless support and belief
in us as our running stories continue to unfold.

To all the worldwide community of runners,
new and experienced, young and old, slow and fast,
including those whose stories are not yet finished.
Keep discovering ways for running to give you
more joy and meaning, and to make your lives complete.

Is something "Ultimately" important to you?
Then we want to know about it. . . .

We hope you enjoyed *The Ultimate Runner*. We are planning many more books in the Ultimate series, each filled with entertaining stories, must-know facts, and captivating photos. We're always looking for talented writers to share slice-of-life true stories, creative photographers to capture images that a story can't tell, as well as top experts to offer their unique insights on a given topic.

For more information on submission guidelines, or to suggest a topic for an upcoming book, please visit the Ultimate website at **www.ultimatehcibooks.com**, or write to: Submission Guidelines, Ultimate Series, HCI Books, 3201 SW 15th St., Deerfield Beach, FL 33442.

For more information about other books by
Health Communications, Inc., please visit **www.hcibooks.com**.

Contents

Introduction

Great moments in running happen every day!

That's our mantra and our deep belief because it has been our actual experience over decades of running. We believe that behind every runner is a story—getting started, a comeback from an injury, a race triumph, or new and rekindled relationships forged through running. Stories about fitness breakthroughs, gritty runs and races, and golden friendships are the fabric of our sport, and we are delighted that so many runners have shared their stories in *The Ultimate Runner*.

We're not talking just about stories of elite runners, Olympians, or even the talented, local champions who win races in our communities each weekend. We're talking about great moments in running among our favorite people, the worldwide community we affectionately call *ordinary runners*. We believe that as ordinary runners we experience great runs, have personal triumphs in races, and achieve life-changing outcomes. Over the years, we have met and talked with countless of ordinary runners who have an *extraordinary* story to tell.

Our favorite stories are more than "race reports." We find wonder and awe in stories about beginning runners in ordinary neighborhoods, including why and how runners got started, how they keep motivated, and how running has changed their lives. We also love stories about running successes and accomplishments. The story may be a training run or a momentous race, returning from a setback, making a lifestyle change, or going faster or farther—or both. We smile at stories about what runners achieve, tingle at what drives them to run, and are in awe of what they've overcome to get there.

We are committed to spreading enthusiasm for running with every runner we meet. We joke, "If you want to lose an hour of your life you'll never get back, just get us talking about running." It's true. We love to hear about others running, what they've accomplished, and what in running they're focusing on at the moment. We know runners run well when they are supported in mind, spirit, and body, and the best support comes from other runners. The collection of stories in *The Ultimate Runner* is our attempt to share some of the best stories and tips as a small way to support runners in our communities.

With the rise of running's popularity, we are also touched to hear stories about charity, community, and support for running and runners. Runners "get it" and are sharing what others in their community are doing for running and the clubs, events, and lives they are touching. In every community there are runners, coaches, businesses, race directors, club leaders, and volunteers who are working tirelessly in ways that impact all of us.

The other joy of working on this book was the privilege of connecting with our experts. While the contributing experts are renowned coaches, accomplished athletes, and leaders in their professions, they have been very approachable, helpful, and interested in sharing sound information with other runners. It's a rare opportunity for ordinary runners like us to work closely with Olympians, national champions, and experts whose work guides and transforms ordinary and elite runners. We believe you will benefit from the expertise they share.

Over the last few years, we have been amazed by how many people tell us, "I'm not really a runner." Some very steady, earnest runners are reluctant to lay claim to the label because running doesn't come easily to them. If they don't run a certain distance— "I just run for 15 to 20 minutes" or a certain frequency, "just a couple times a week," or haven't reached a milestone, "I've only run a couple 5Ks,"—they don't feel entitled to call themselves runners. Nonsense!

We are determined to squelch that mind-set and to outlaw the words *I'm not a runner*. We encourage every runner to see the importance and right to proclaim himself or herself a runner. We believe no matter what the distance, speed, or race acclaim, everyone who gets out there is a runner and a bona fide part of the running community. We believe every runner in some way advances our sport.

Inspiring stories about running deserve a special place where others can enjoy and be uplifted by them. *The Ultimate Runner* is that place. It is a treasury of stories and photos that expresses what running means and how it transforms lives. It is a collection that we hope will continue to motivate you and will inspire you to press toward your own running goals. Every runner has a story to share, including those stories that are not finished yet.

Running races, breaking records, and earning new PRs advance our sport. But more important, our amazing stories are formed when we take time out of our busy lives, get out the door in our ordinary neighborhoods, and reaffirm that great moments in running happen every day!

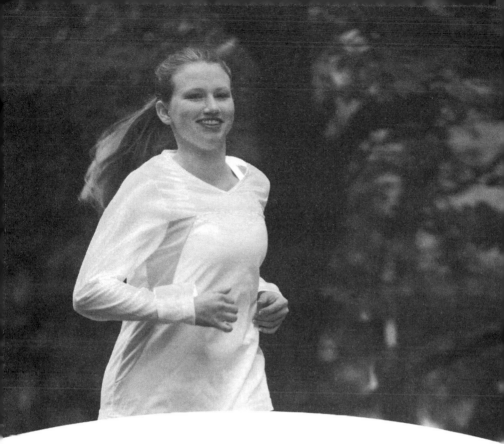

Why We Run:
Physical Transformation

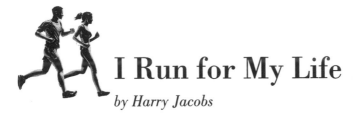

I Run for My Life

by Harry Jacobs

People often ask me "Why do you run?" My answer is quick and to the point: "I run for my life." Usually that gets a snicker and a snide comment about being chased by muggers. But, honestly, I run because if I didn't run, I would be on my way to a heart attack or a stroke.

In May 2005, at the age of forty-seven, I was at the doctor's office for a follow-up after my physical. I stared at the doctor who told me I was being diagnosed with type 2 diabetes. He explained that if I did not change my ways, I would be dead before I was sixty.

I had recently connected with the most wonderful woman in the world, so when I realized my choices were to either shape up or be carried out in a pine box, I knew I had to get serious. So after a brief discussion about meds, the doctor agreed to give me a month to lose weight and get my blood sugar under control.

I jumped on the freight scale at work; my weight was 297 pounds, and it was clear that I had my work cut out for me. I had been a runner back in high school and into my twenties, so I decided that running would be the exercise of choice. Of course, because I hadn't exercised for thirty years, I started out slowly. I was so slow in fact, that my kids would often walk beside me as I huffed and puffed around the block. Soon though, I was jogging for ten minutes a day, adding one minute a week along with frequent walks during my work and lunch breaks. Exercising for forty to sixty minutes a day, I coupled this with a 1400–1600 calorie diet that was recommended by the American Diabetes Association.

My girlfriend (who is now my wife) would often join me during my lunchtime walks. She was very supportive of my diet and exercise plan. When I jumped on the freight scale at the end of the first week, I'd lost one pound. I was also watching my blood glucose levels like a hawk, and soon my diet and exercise brought my blood sugar under control.

When I returned to the doctor at the end of the first month, I was down to 289 pounds and my glucose levels were better. He determined that as long as I stayed on track I could forgo medications.

Changing one life is not easy. Choosing strict control for my blood sugar meant that I had to mimic normal blood sugar levels, which meant changing my eating habits to smaller, more nutrient-dense foods from the typical three big meals a day plus snacks. I became aware of how foods work together to make you feel full even if you eat less. It became about making healthy choices every day.

It was tough watching folks eat sugar-filled foods that I loved—ice cream, cake, and candy, not to mention all those great foods laden with carbohydrates such as bagels, muffins, and pasta. Now life came down to do choosing between a half a slice of bread or an apple, and balancing my meals properly to maximize, not only the calories, but the nutrients needed to keep me active and healthy.

At the end of three months, my fasting blood sugar was in the normal range, I was twenty pounds lighter, and I was running between twenty and thirty minutes a day. I still moved slowly, but I was moving and I could see signs of fitness. Going up and down stairs was much easier. There was a bounce in my step, and I was feeling stronger physically.

In March, one of my colleagues at work told me about the Scotiabank Blue Nose Marathon. Even though by this time I was running more, I scoffed at the idea of running a marathon. But later, I thought about it and finally told myself, *I can do this*. The next week I registered for the 10K event that was also being run that day.

At that point I was running seven to eight kilometers, and I knew I had time to get my distance up to the 10K mark. While I was out running one Sunday a group of runners went by me going in the opposite direction. It turned out that they were part of a local running club and ran every Sunday morning with varied distances depending on the event. As it turned out, they had a group training for the Blue Nose 10K event. The next week I was at the club with everyone else, which turned out to be a life-changing event. I was not just running by myself but with a group of like-minded people, each one running for his or her own reason, but at the same time giving support to each other. Over the next weeks our distance slowly crossed the 10K mark up to 14K two weeks before the race. There was no question now about running 10K—it was in the bag.

On the day of my first 10K race, I happened to be introduced to John Stanton, the CEO of the Running Room. When he asked me if I was running the marathon, my reply was "No, just the 10K." What he told me stays with me to this day. He looked me in the eye, told me I was not *just* running a 10K; this was my race, I trained for it, and I should not diminish its importance. He went on to tell me I was an athlete, which made me laugh as I never considered myself an athlete in any way. Again he explained that the moment I strapped on my running shoes I became a runner. Speed was not important; it was the activity and going the distance that mattered. Then he made me laugh by saying it was not how fast I ran, but how good I looked at the end for the finish-line photograph.

I finished that 10K race in just under sixty-four minutes, well under the seventy-minute goal I set for myself. That year I also went on to run a half marathon in 2:06 and became an instructor teaching a Running Room Learn to Run Clinic. After one year I had dropped a total of eighty-six pounds and was a far cry from that guy who was barely able to walk around the block. I can tell you, I looked very good.

Running saved my life—it forever changed me. I am not the same person I was, neither physically nor mentally. Not only did I change my life, but I went on and gave back to the sport I learned to love, teaching others not only to run but giving them the tools to change their lives, too. Running, I learned, is not just exercise: it is a lifestyle.

Fast forward another three years: I am fifty-one years old, a veteran runner, and my weight is stable at 208 pounds. I still run five to six days a week and run races when I can. My current doctor would not know I was a diabetic because none of my tests show any signs of the disease and I continue to be medication-free. I run for my life and will continue to do so right up to the day they put me in that pine box. Which I hope will not be for a long while yet!

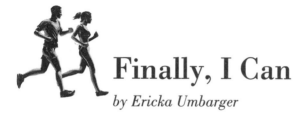

Finally, I Can

by Ericka Umbarger

In April 1993, I was thirteen years old when I was diagnosed with polyarticular juvenile rheumatoid arthritis in every single joint in my body. Within a matter of weeks, I went from a very physical, active child who participated in basketball, running, gymnastics, volleyball, and softball, to one who could barely get out of bed and walk the halls of school. My body easily felt like that of an eighty-year-old. Once the fastest girl at the school (and actually faster than most of the boys), I now had to sit on the sidelines and watch everyone in gym class; my knees, hands, shoulders, hips, and elbows were too swollen to allow me to play. When my middle-school class went on a field trip to a roller-skating rink, I wasn't allowed to go because I might fall and hurt myself. Instead, I had to stay at school and catch up with my school work.

The ten years after my diagnosis are a blur, and to be honest, I've blocked a lot of it out. If I thought middle school was tough, high school was worse. High school consisted of fighting for accommodations in my classrooms, using the elevator at school instead of stairs, and being homeschooled when my ankles were too swollen for me to walk. I missed more than twenty days one year and was threatened with failing, despite maintaining an A/B average in all my classes. I couldn't hang out with friends on the weekends because I was in so much pain, and I felt even more awkward because of my limp and because of the weight gain from steroids. I suffered from anorexia for one year and bulimia for almost seven years, going to extreme measures to gain some sort of control in my life.

College consisted of many of the same problems, but thankfully I had surrounded myself with a more supportive group. My arthritis, though still painful and active, became tolerable, and I was able to take a backpacking course—that made me fall in love with the outdoors all over again. And in the past fourteen years, I've had thirteen surgeries to help correct some of the deformities in my hands.

Fast forward to 2003. Besides the anti-inflammatory medication and oral chemotherapy I was taking for my arthritis, I became financially eligible to begin taking a self-injectible biologic drug. Within weeks of taking this weekly shot, I ran my first 5K in November 2003: the Arthritis Foundation's Jingle Bell Run/ Walk, and I finished just under thirty minutes. I was determined that it would not stop there. My goal was to train for a 10K in April 2004; I turned my training into a self-improvement project for a graduate school class I was taking for my master of social work degree. Then came the half marathons in April and September 2005 and April 2006. At that point, I dared to let myself believe that I may actually be able to run a marathon.

On a whim, I signed up for my first marathon to be run in November 2006, not really knowing for sure if I would be able to do it. I trained for almost five months with the Sports Backers Marathon Training Team in Richmond, Virginia, and things were going well . . . until three and a half weeks before my marathon. I was diagnosed with a stress fracture in the pubic ramus (pelvic area) and was told the injury itself would take six to nine weeks to recover from, and then I could start running again. However, I was likely to miss the marathon—my sole focus of the last five months—as my doctor gave me only a 25 percent chance of recovery by marathon morning. I'd already had running taken away from me for ten years; I was determined not to let it happen again. I realized I could give up then and regret not trying to achieve my dream, or I could fight a good fight and give it all I had.

For the next three weeks I cross-trained for three hours every day, tracked my pain levels, met with my doctors, and decided that even if I had to walk the whole thing, I would be crossing that finish line. I refused to have my dream taken away from me again. That morning, I think I was so full of adrenaline I didn't even feel the pain until mile sixteen, at which point I had to start walking and then ran/walked the last ten miles. Even so, afflicted with juvenile rheumatoid arthritis and injured with a stress fracture, I still managed to finish my first marathon in 4:09:18.

And it definitely didn't stop there. In the past two and a half years, I've run a total of seven marathons with a personal record (PR) of 3:53:38. In January 2008, just a few months before my twenty-eighth birthday, I decided to push myself even farther and started doing ultramarathons. Since then, I've completed four 50Ks, one forty-miler, and two fifty-milers, including a 50K on April 26, 2008 that was only three weeks after I had three joints in my hands completely replaced (surgery number thirteen). My goal is to eventually run the Umstead 100-Mile Endurance Run in North Carolina and use it as a fund-raising opportunity for the Arthritis Foundation. I am far from the fastest runner out there, but I am one of the most thankful and have more drive and determination than most since running was taken from me for so long.

My running comes at a price. Besides the weekly oral chemotherapy, I also have a four-hour infusion every six weeks at the hospital, weekly shots, and blood tests every six weeks to monitor liver and kidney functions. My doctors do not fully understand my passion and determination, but they fully support my decision to continue living my dream. They know that to keep me from running would kill my spirit.

Sixteen years ago, I was told that one day I might not be able to walk and would spend the rest of my life in a wheelchair. I spent so many years believing this that I forgot to believe in myself. So when people ask me why I run, I simply tell them that it is because . . . finally, I can.

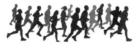

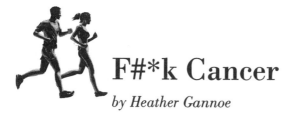

F#*k Cancer

by Heather Gannoe

My story is really "Her Story," but her story tells the tale of how I was inspired to become a runner.

It was February 2005. Months earlier, my loving and crazy older sister had somehow convinced my younger sister and me to run the Myrtle Beach Dasani Half Marathon with her. Thinking it was no biggie, and we'd have plenty of time to train, we said yes. Well, working, partying, and other more important things (hey, I was a twenty-three-year-old living in a vacation town) got in the way, and I don't believe I had run but, oh, maybe a mile or two on the treadmill the week prior to the race. Race morning came, I donned my two-and-a-half-year-old worn-out Nikes, and took my place at the start corral. I had no idea what I was in for.

To spare you a pathetic story, it sucked. I couldn't walk for a week. But darn it, I finished that stupid half marathon, and I still have the medal and pictures to prove it. I couldn't understand why anyone would put themselves through that kind of misery, never mind jump at any chance they could to register for a race, like Holly was always doing.

That afternoon, lying on my couch in misery and pain, Holly

said she had something to tell us. Recently, she had noticed a spot on her back that was new and questionable. She had been to the doctor already, but after the race would return home for some more testing. But we shouldn't have to worry. So, I didn't—until I got a phone call about a week later. Holly had been diagnosed with an aggressive form of cancer, stage 3 nodular melanoma.

At the time of diagnosis, Holly had a calendar full of races, including the Marine Corps Marathon that fall. She now had to add two major surgeries to remove the cancer and some lymph nodes, as well as four weeks of high-dose chemotherapy, followed by forty-eight more weeks of low-dose chemotherapy. But in true Holly fashion, this did not deter her from her goals. Holly continued training for the marathon.

That fall, I joined Holly to run the 2005 Army Ten-Miler. I was still not a runner, and the race still sucked for me. You would have thought the half marathon had taught me a lesson, but I am a bit stubborn and hardheaded. Needless to say, I struggled. As anyone who may have run the 2005 Army Ten-Miler will remember, a bomb threat at a bridge on the racecourse resulted in a detour, which resulted in the race becoming the "Army 11.4-Miler." It was a little confusing toward the end, as no one on the course had any idea where we were going, what was going on, or how much farther we had to go. None of the volunteers on the side of the road would utter anything other than "just keep going." But Holly had reached the end of her rope and started to break down. The confusion, the exhaustion, the uncertainty—it had all gotten to her. The pale look on her face and knowing what her body was going through terrified me at that moment. Should we even be out there?

But we pushed each other through, and as we finally crossed a bridge toward the finish line, Holly screamed out "F#*K CAN-CER!!!" I have never in my entire life been so moved or in awe of another human being as I was at that moment. There I was, feeling downright sorry for myself, struggling to finish a race when I would have preferred to be in bed. And there was Holly, her body worn and broken down from months and months of chemotherapy, and she was running, giving every last drop of energy she could muster up, and she was happy to be doing it. I felt selfish. Selfish for taking my body for granted. And amazed at my beautiful sister and her strength.

From that moment on, I wanted to be a runner. I wanted to be as proud of my body and accomplishments as my sister was of hers. I wanted to be just like my hero.

On October 30, 2005, Holly "beat the 14th Street Bridge" and successfully finished the Marine Corps Marathon. She continued on with six more months of chemotherapy treatment and successfully beat cancer.

She also managed to successfully turn her little sister into a running junkie. Since that race, I have run countless more races of all different distances, many of them with Holly by my side. But I wasn't the only one she would have that effect on. Holly later founded the Cancer to 5K Training Program, with the help and support of the Ulman Cancer Fund for Young Adults. Holly and her team of volunteers help coach other young adult cancer patients and survivors to become runners and complete their first 5K.

She is making a difference in the lives of everyone she comes in contact with. In my eyes, she is nothing short of amazing. Thank you, Holly. I love you!

How the Great Wall Changed My Life

by Brian Aldrich

I had just finished my sophomore year of college in 2005 when I went to visit my parents for the summer. They had been living in China for a year and this was my first trip there. The Chinese said I looked like Buddha, and the shirtmakers loved me because I need a lot of fabric for my shirts, thus driving the price up. I was five feet ten and more than 290 pounds; I knew I was a big kid, and I embraced it even though I wasn't healthy. When September came and it was time for me to return to college, I remember tearing up, thinking about how lucky I was to be standing on the Great Wall of China. I never thought I'd be back. Little did I know this trip was only the beginning.

I stepped on the scale when I was back at school, and it read "err"—which meant I was over 300 pounds. I'd let my weight get out of hand. I'd told myself that if I ever saw "300" I would start to do something about it, so that very day I stopped drinking soda, which was my lifeblood, and started planning to get into shape.

I remember my father going out for runs with his buddies when I was young. It seemed to keep him in shape, but I didn't understand how getting out the door and running could be any fun. But if he liked it, I thought I would give it a try. The next day, I started jogging. I picked a spot to run to from my dorm only half a mile away, but I couldn't make it halfway there without walking. Maybe it was the cold, or the fact I was about 300 pounds, but it was brutal. Over the next month, I progressed from walking most of the way to jogging part of it, to running both directions, and eventually I did my first full mile as a runner.

People started to notice the change in my appearance. I started getting compliments and didn't know how to accept them; it was new for me to be told how good I looked. The more compliments I received, the more I ran and the better my diet became. It took me a year to get to two miles. I was *very* overweight to start, so motivation came and went over the first year; this wasn't a fast-paced *Biggest Loser* story.

A week or so after running my first two-mile stretch, I was on the Great Wall again. The Wall had witnessed a transformation —I was about thirty pounds lighter than I'd been a year earlier. I thought *this* would be my last time on the Wall, but again I didn't know what was to come.

When I returned home, my mom encouraged me to start training for my first 10K. The thought of running a race had always been in the back of my head, but a race had never seemed achievable. I started running longer distances—three miles here, four miles there. By now, I loved running. I was still uncomfortable running in the gym because of my weight, so I tried as best I could to stay outside and work on the terrain. In March 2007, I ran my first 10K with my mom. As a kid you always know how much your mother loves you, but actually seeing the look on her face as she saw me finish my first race was a great feeling. That race was a real turning point for me; I craved more races and started blogging about my running. The community of online running bloggers provided a wealth of knowledge money can't buy. These were real people trading war stories about running. With every post I wrote and read, my desire to run increased. I had the itch: I was a runner.

Over the next year I completed eight other races, including three half marathons, two 5Ks, two more 10Ks, and a six-miler. I finished every race the same way—by applauding myself for a job well done.

I literally ran 100 pounds off my body in that year. It all happened so fast. I loved to run and no longer was worried about my weight-loss journey. I knew I would become much healthier with every run. I just wanted to run. At Christmastime in 2008, I told my parents I wanted to train for my first marathon, but I wanted to make my first one count. To me, a marathon would be the Super Bowl of the racing world. Marathons aren't for everyone, but this was something I wanted to achieve. And I decided the perfect race to be my first marathon would be the 2009 Great Wall Marathon.

I spent eighteen weeks training for this not-so-typical first marathon. I encountered many "mile"stones as I trained; I ran distances I never thought were reachable, even calling my parents halfway around the world and bragging when I reached my first fifteen. I trained on the parking garage staircase. My legs had to be at their strongest as this race would be a true endurance test.

"You're doing what?" friends and family would ask me. They

didn't believe me when I told them I was actually going to run on the Great Wall. I learned a lot about my mental and physical health in those eighteen weeks, and sooner than I could ever imagine I was on a flight to Beijing. This was to be the biggest event of my life. One hundred and twenty pounds ago I'd never dreamed I could run a marathon, yet here I was, on my way!

The marathon course was split into three chunks. The race started with five swerving uphill kilometers to the entrance of the two-mile stretch of the Great Wall. This two-mile stretch of wall was 10 percent runable. It included towers, upward ladder-style staircases, and a couple of goat paths; a true endurance test. There were parts to the Wall with only one side, making it impossible for anyone to pass without the risk of falling straight down. Some of these death traps had railings or ropes, and some had nothing. After rushing through that, we were back in the square where the race began and had fifteen miles around the villages. Once we returned from the fifteen, we ran the reverse of the first five miles.

My parents, who had also signed up for the race, encouraged me to run my own race, so I did. I split off early and just got in my groove. I caught up with my dad at mile sixteen as he was starting mile thirteen. This was his tenth marathon, and being able to hug him at my first marathon was amazing. We were running the same race; I am sure he never thought I would be running in a marathon with him.

As I was coming into the starting area again I heard people cheering me on, and my mom was running up to me. "You're going to do it!" she yelled as I nearly started to tear up. She had run the 10K portion of the race and was able to see me enter the

Wall for the second time. With another kiss and a hug, I headed toward the starting area to get up on the Wall. I was doing well, I knew that.

As I reached the top of one of the towers I began to see the harsh reality of this marathon. People were lying on the Wall, backs against it, completely drained of all energy, some shaking their heads and some sponging their heads to cool down. I couldn't let this get to me. The second time through the Wall was scary, but I had to run my own race. I raced into the square and started clapping, my signature move—this time it meant much more. I raced through the finish line and landed on the mat at 5:36:40.

I had done it. I'd run my first marathon. As soon as the medal was around my neck, my mom hugged me. She was probably still crying from the previous time she'd seen me.

The Great Wall wasn't the end of my journey; it was the beginning of two journeys. It kicked off my weight loss in 2005 and later, it became my first marathon. It was the hardest thing I have ever done—and I wouldn't have chosen another marathon as my first. Coming from 300 pounds to 180 pounds *and* running my first marathon *with* my parents was the ride of a lifetime. Running changed my life, and it all began with the Great Wall of China.

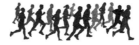

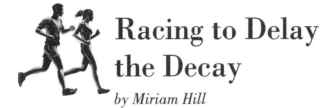

Racing to Delay the Decay

by Miriam Hill

I t is two hours past midnight, the weather is sultry, and I'm sopping wet as I walk among the hundreds of tired runners after finishing the 3K race in the annual Fourth of July Kiwinis Morton Plant Mease Midnight Run in Dunedin, Florida. We're physically drained, and we munch on bananas, gulp Gatorade, and wait for the race results. My heart leaps when I hear my name over the loudspeaker. Applause fills my ears as I step forward to receive my plaque. The printing reads: THIRD PLACE, WOMEN'S, 60–64 3K. As I beam with pride, a trim, young woman approaches me.

"I tried to catch you throughout the race, but I couldn't. Well done!"

Her words are as rewarding as the plaque.

I was in my late thirties when one evening I decided to go jogging. After one block I was winded, but I stuck with it and made progress as I ran some more. During the next few months I continued to run and increased my distance and speed. As my body grew stronger, I knew that running was the exercise I wanted to incorporate into my life. There were other athletes in my family; my husband was a dedicated runner and my daughters ran cross-country on their high school teams.

But having a middle-aged mom show interest in running was unexpected. I set a goal that on my fortieth birthday I would run four miles. My best birthday present was accomplishing that goal. As I continued to build my endurance, I began to enter races.

The largest race in my area is the Turkey Trot, held on Thanksgiving Day in Clearwater, Florida. More than 10,000 people run this race before they sit down to Thanksgiving dinner. One year when my children were young, the *St. Petersburg Times* published a picture and front-page story about our family, because my husband and I were running the Turkey Trot with our three children. Now that the kids are grown they have fond memories of those Thanksgiving races.

"Mom, I don't know how you did it!" says Betsy. "You would always run the Turkey Trot with us and afterward Thanksgiving dinner would magically appear on the table! I can hardly get my dinner ready . . . without running a race first!"

As my fiftieth birthday approached, I kept running to "delay the decay" of aging. The day I turned fifty I ran five miles. When I turned sixty-three, I signed up for the 10K race at Disney World. I had to do my best since officials promised to pick up slow runners and remove them from the competition. Being hauled off in a Mickey Mouse mobile would be embarrassing.

When I finally crossed the finish line, I heard my name over the loudspeaker and received congratulations for completing the Disney World 10K Classic. I have a certificate from Disney that reads, *Congratulations! You've conquered The World on Foot.*

My race time didn't shatter any records, but it was a victory for my aging body that's . . . racing to delay the decay.

Never Give Up: My Journey to Become a Runner

by Bridgette L. Collins

I'm glad it's okay to bring the past to life from time to time. Those periodic reflections remind me how I emerged from an unhealthy time period in my life. Gripped in toxic lifestyle habits, fractured relationships, and a lack of self-love, my perspective of the things that really mattered was out of focus. I often thought, *If only I could change the way I look and feel, my life could be different.* It was a nice thought, but it needed to be combined with action. My life is richer today because of God's plan to free me and help me focus my attention. Little did I know, though, His plan for a healthy mind, body, and spirit would involve running.

It was the summer of 1994, but I remember the conversation as though it were yesterday. I had started sharing with a group of coworkers my discontent with working out at the gym on the StairMaster, stationary bike, and circuit machinery. After three weeks of alternating between the machines and changing my routine several times, I was discouraged by a lack of physical changes. I carried layers of excess body fat, and I was looking for and expecting instant results for my efforts.

Ken, my supervisor, walked into the break room and joined the conversation. "Maybe you'd enjoy an outside activity better. Have you ever thought about running?" he asked me.

A voice inside my head put up a defense. *What is he talking about? Running! Not interested. I'm not going to exert that kind of energy.*

As Ken eagerly shared his passion for running through the hilly neighborhoods of Huntsville, Texas, I interrupted him with a friendly smile and said, "That's not an activity I'm interested in."

From that day forward, though, every time I saw Ken, he would ask, "Have you started running yet? I have a hunch you'll really like it." Each time, he'd have a different running story to share with me. But I was more interested in hearing about quick and easy solutions for losing unwanted body fat rather than hearing his whirlwind of running stories.

My responses were always filled with an array of excuses. I kept thinking of aching body parts. Perhaps it was the visions of that chubby kid in middle school forced to run around a track that still haunted me, or thoughts of sweat streaming down my face, ruining my makeup, and stirring up acne-prone skin, or the amount of time I'd need afterward to restore my hair to its stylish look. No, running did not fit into my plans. I was looking for fun, easy, and low-maintenance solutions. Running sounded harsh, painful, and time-consuming.

But as time passed, I was inspired more and more by Ken's stories. He talked about logging forty to fifty miles each week, his training experiences, and running marathons, all of which sounded foreign to me. But after one conversation, I thought perhaps I could run on the treadmill at the gym. That would be a good way to get started, and I could always quit if I didn't like it.

A week later, I started my regimen of walking thirty to forty minutes on the treadmill. As I attempted to increase my speed, I would become winded and I tired easily. I contemplated giving up as I observed others, younger and smaller in size, running with ease and comfort. I thought to myself, *I'll never get it. This whole idea is a mistake.*

I shared my frustration with Ken one day. "All I feel is discouragement and disappointment when I see younger women running so easily and confidently on the treadmill," I lamented. "Why can't it be like that for me? Maybe running isn't for me. Maybe I'm too big."

Sensing my doubts and fears, he responded in a quiet voice, "First, let me say that runners come in different shapes and sizes. Second, two things you need to succeed at anything are desire and commitment. You are my top recruiter and I know firsthand that you have both qualities. There could be a number of reasons why you tire easily. Keep in mind this is a new activity for you." He proceeded to give me some strategies for building my endurance. He stressed the importance of eating the right foods at the right times during the day, staying hydrated, wearing appropriate footwear and apparel, and learning to pace my steps.

Perhaps my biggest challenge was eating right. That was the one thing I had never really addressed. As I started researching the foods I had come to rely on for comfort, I recognized that some of my eating habits had to change. *This is going to be hard*, I thought one day after reading the labels for some of my favorite foods. *Everything I love to eat is lacking in the vital nutrients Ken talked about. They are loaded with salt, sugar, and transfats.* My discoveries prompted me to figure out how to make my favorite foods healthier and more beneficial to my body. For me, it also meant no more all-you-can-eat buffets. No more guzzling two cans of my favorite soda each day. No more scarfing down cookies, chips, and candy bars. No more nachos and cheese fries. No more happy hour!

"Always think progression," Ken pointed out in the same quiet voice. "Above all, visualize yourself running with confidence and ease. You can achieve what you visualize and pursue. That's why I like running marathons. They force me to push my body to the next level and beyond its comfort zone. And when you think about it, that's the way we should live our lives—always ready to push ourselves to the next level."

I embraced Ken's words of encouragement, determined to become a runner. I executed a workout program that included an array of strength-building and flexibility exercises to complement my time on the treadmill. I went to the gym most days, and over a period of time, my endurance and aerobic capacity improved. Tales of Ken's passion for running remained in the back of my mind and helped me overcome my insecurities. And yes, the inevitable did happen. I sweated heavily during my runs. My hair became drenched. My acne-prone skin was irritated. But I figured out how to lessen the impact: I kept a towel by my side to wipe my face, I got a new hairstyle more conducive to exercise, and I was prescribed an acne medication. I was on my on my way to becoming a true runner!

After several weeks of running on the treadmill, I upgraded to a community track in Huntsville. I headed there most days after work. As my endurance increased, I added a lap or so each week. To my surprise, I actually looked forward to running around that track while listening to fast tunes on my cassette player. All along, I was shedding excess body fat day by day, week by week. But something extraordinary was also happening. For the first time in my life, I was able to focus with vigilance, confidence, and passion on the things that really mattered. After each run, I thought, *Wow! Is this what it feels like to be happy and free?*

My newfound passion for running around that track brought me to a place I had never experienced. It was apparent that God used running to help focus my attention and prepare me for a journey. It was the place where I found the solitude to pinpoint why I allowed situations to create unhealthy thoughts, attitudes, and actions. Those laps around the track produced solutions for change that led me to redefine my limits.

I'm a better person and in a better position because of the decisions I made and the actions I took during the summer of 1994. Running has transformed my body, mind, and soul. Sure, I've endured sore muscles, scraped knees, tight hamstrings, shin splints, plantar fasciitis—all the pain and discomfort of a runner—but no matter what, running helped me reevaluate my life. It freed me to discover my potential and gave me the desire to live generously.

Through the completion of four marathons, a wealth of training, and the creation of my own company focused on helping others to live more healthfully, my life is now filled with purpose and peace. Running was part of God's plan to elevate me to a position where I could make a difference in the lives of others, like Ken made in mine. I am so glad I didn't give up!

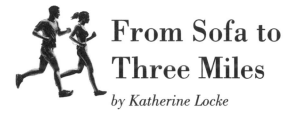

From Sofa to Three Miles

by Katherine Locke

I t's a very early morning in May and I am running through town. Last year at this time, I was so sick I could barely walk down the stairs. And now here I am running. I was diagnosed with breast cancer in February 2007, and ten grueling months of treatment followed; I had two rounds of surgery, five months of chemotherapy, followed by fifteen sessions of radiotherapy. I emerged from it all just before Christmas, weak, totally unfit, and twenty-eight pounds overweight.

The ten months of treatment aged me by ten years. My hair is thin and my weight gain makes me look (and feel) dowdy and middle-aged. I was so sick during the chemotherapy that there were days I couldn't stand upright. The steroids I took after each session to help with the nausea puffed me up beyond recognition. They also made me ravenously hungry. For two or three days after each chemo, the nausea meant that nothing, or dry toast, was all I could keep down.

Then the steroids would kick in and I would be so hungry I could have eaten my own arm. It was a mad, crazed hunger I couldn't control, and I couldn't stop thinking about food. Everything tasted delicious, and bread was my biggest weakness. Meals were so huge and with so many courses that they merged into one another until I was eating all day. The pounds piled on.

I can't blame all my weight gain on the cancer treatment, however. I was already overweight and desperately unfit. Up to 8 percent of breast-cancer cases are attributed to being overweight. As my health deteriorated, my lifestyle slowed down to a spectacularly sedentary pace. Being unfit before diagnosis undoubtedly made going through the treatment process more difficult. Cancer fatigue and physical impairment is suffered by 70 percent of people going through chemotherapy, and I was badly afflicted. By the time it was all over I was desperate to get fit, but had no idea where to start. I was still so very weak and my confidence so low that the thought of going to the gym was horrifying.

I decided to hire a personal trainer. I needed someone who would understand my particular circumstances and give me an individually tailored exercise schedule. This wasn't the cheapest option, but I instinctively knew it is the right thing to do. Some people want to book a fabulous holiday, or have regular massage sessions after a cancer diagnosis; in my case, I felt that rest wasn't best—I needed to learn how to move again.

My wonderful trainer gave me exactly what I needed. She suggested I enter the Race for Life (a three-mile race to raise money for cancer research in the UK) and I dismissed it out of hand. *How can I even think about running when I can barely walk?* Then I thought again. *What a sense of achievement if I manage to run it! It's four months away. Can I possibly do it? I haven't run since I was a child.* I checked out the website and was inspired by the sheer numbers—35,000 women who'd had personal experiences with cancer. I decided to sign up, and even if I had to walk, it was something to aim for.

The first time I tried to run in my training, I manage to stumble about 200 yards before collapsing with exhaustion. I found a track that was about 400 yards. It took weeks to be strong enough to make it around one time. I started to run every other day, building up each session by one minute each time, until I could run for ten minutes without stopping, which was three times around the track.

I kept up my running religiously. There were days when I exceeded my goals and days when I didn't. The weight started to shift slowly, almost imperceptibly at first, at a steady rate of about one pound per week. Ironically, running made me want to eat less, not more, and I began to regulate my food intake back to normal levels. I was starting to regain my strength, and my confidence was coming back. I was getting into clothes I hadn't worn for a long time, and I began to feel the benefits of regular exercise, such as more energy and a better mood.

Then a month before the race I hit a wall. The farthest I had managed to run was just under two miles, split into walk/run intervals. I really suffered after the exertion and endured aching legs and numb tiredness that reminded me of my chemo days. I was worried. My running high had evaporated and my hips hurt— a lot. I'd read that chemotherapy drugs can adversely affect joints, and suddenly I wondered if it was crazy to attempt to run so far after everything I'd been through. Was it mad to choose now to get fit, after a cancer diagnosis?

I started to research statistics about exercising after cancer and was astounded to discover that regular exercise can cut the risk of secondary cancers by up to 50 percent. That's more effective than some drug therapies. But while there have been studies proving the beneficial effects of exercise going back as far as the early 1990s, finding anything but the most general advice on how to start exercising after treatment was very difficult.

I uncovered research from the *British Medical Journal* that proved aerobic exercise is particularly valuable and has long-term positive effects. This was the spur I needed, and I dragged myself out again—through slow, steady running, my time and distance increased by tiny increments, sometimes only seconds, each time. The race was my goal. As I trained, I visualized myself running the actual race and enjoying the sense of achievement I would feel.

The week preceding the race was damp and cool and perfect for running, and I managed a couple of good runs that boosted my confidence. I had been praying for cool weather, as running in the heat was particularly difficult. Tamoxifen (the drug I will be taking for the next five years) can impair the body's ability to regulate temperature and I am permanently hot. The day of the race was blisteringly hot, though. I was anxious and also concerned about the crowds. The Race for Life is extremely popular, with events all over the UK. My local race had more than 2,000 women participating. The cancer experience is a very solitary one, and I hadn't been in a large crowd for a long time. All I could make out as I arrived was a sea of pink. There were groups of women of all shapes and sizes, families on picnic blankets—a festival atmosphere. Lots of runners wore tags on their back with the names of people who have been affected by cancer. It was tremendously moving, and during the warm-up I felt tears begin.

But there was no time for sentiment because suddenly we were off. As I ran I realized I could do this. Many women were walking and chatting, but I really wanted to run. The heat and bottlenecks were against us, but I could do it. I could run three miles!

I came in with a respectable time of forty-four minutes. It wasn't going to break any records, but from where I'd come from, I felt like a world champion.

Will I enter the race again? I'm not sure. Will I stop running? Not on your life. My sofa days are behind me.

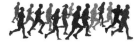

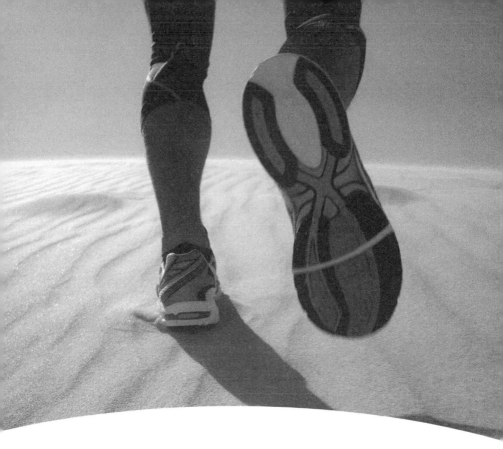

Emotional and
Spiritual Insights

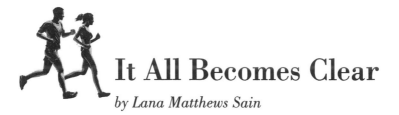

It All Becomes Clear

by Lana Matthews Sain

I have come to the conclusion that there is not too much in life that a good twenty-mile run can't fix. Make that a twenty-mile run in the fall, when it's cool but not cold. The air is crisp but not dry. The sun rises and shines brightly, but it does not scorch. The wind swirls but it does not rage against your momentum.

In the course of the three hours and three minutes it took me to cover twenty miles on foot this morning, I reviewed the past three or four weeks of aimless wandering and struggling to find purpose in the many miles I've volunteered to put my body through. I miraculously regained the focus and zoned clearly in on the goal. I saw it. I fixed my eyes on it, and I remembered why this was such a worthy goal in the first place.

The Ironman competition is not some current line item being checked off my "bucket list." I'm not "doin' it to say I did." I'm not doing it for the M-Dot ink (the official Ironman logo). I'm not doing it for recognition or acceptance. I'm not even trying to inspire you; or my kids.

Do you really want to know why I'm out there? Why I chose to go all in, to bet it all and sign my 2008 life away to a one-day event in November? Why I get up at 3:00 AM and run in the dark? Why I drop the kids off at school and ride my bike until it's time to pick them up again, and why I slip back out of the house at 8:00 PM to get the swim in before bedtime?

Because I have learned that if you don't actively take a stand against it, the nature of the world will ever so slightly dull your senses, soften your will, and limit your amazing, natural-born capacity. It will lie to you. It will beat you down. You will forget who you are, and at the time you least expect it, it will throw you a curveball it knows you won't be able to hit. You won't see the beauty of the sunrise because you'll be asleep. You won't feel the stillness of night because you'll be engrossed in reality television. You'll opt out of that game of tag with the little one because you can't catch your breath. You won't take a risk, because you might fail. You won't enter the event because you might not win. You won't consider the unthinkable because *You Are Just Average*. You will lose the magnificence and beauty, the combination of uniqueness and grandeur that the Creator formed you with in His own image. You will walk the rest of your days on the earth wondering who you are and why you are here. You will stand on the sidelines and hide from the coach when you think he's about to call your number to go in the game. You won't experience the pain of coming up one second short, but you also won't feel the exhilaration of coming back against all odds. You might not get knocked down or skinned up, but you won't know the gratification of pulling yourself back up and finishing with respect. You won't ever know what you could've done or who you could've been.

I knew that the journey to Ironman would strip me of the unnecessary baggage I clutter my life with, and it would get all up in my face to show me again who I really am. I knew that it would force me to shut up for once, to stop complaining and stop making excuses and just watch, listen, and learn. Somewhere amid the neurons in my subconscious, I knew that I would be left with no other choice but to accept that "I praise you because I am fearfully and wonderfully made; your works are wonderful, I know that full well." (Psalms 139:14 NIV) Whatever it takes that I may be able to spend my days on this earth in celebration and appreciation of this truth, I will do it.

Ironman, you are mine.

Breaking
Your Own Tape

by Marcia Puryear

How many times have we watched in awe and amazement as the elites seem to fly through the finish line of a marathon; arms held high in some primal feeling of supreme satisfaction, pure fulfillment, relief, and perhaps shear but blissful exhaustion? How must it feel to touch that shiny band of ultimate victory that stretches taut across the end of the course—to be the first runner, the only runner, to feel it snap and break against your chest? The touch of victory? The ultimate "high five" from the gods of champions? The very first tangible, palpable acknowledgment of having done a job and done it well?

We merely mortal, but just as passionate, runners can do the same thing. Every one of us has our own finish-line tape. In our minds, we have each formulated our own goal for this mission: to simply finish feeling strong, to cut time from our last marathon, a PR, or to quietly honor a cause or person who needs support. Our tape is personal, woven from the fabric of our dreams, our reality, and our own truth. Breaking our symbolic tape can be an incredibly meaningful moment—physically, emotionally, and spiritually.

No matter what our skill level might be, this is where we share a common spirit with the elites. No matter whether we attempt a two-hour run or one that is more than five hours, we all can own that gut-level feeling of pure, honest achievement and fulfillment. We can have this complete acknowledgment of our own job well done. As marathon runner and author John Bingham wrote in his book *Marathoning for Mortals*, "Your spirit doesn't know how to tell time."

So you did it. You broke your own personal tape, the tape that marks the completion of your mission. No matter how it hurt, no matter that you had moments of doubt, fear, thoughts of giving up, no matter even if you changed your goal midrace. Your mind managed the demons that can destroy you. You stayed focused on your mission, your mind's eye always keen on the runner within you, keeping you positive, alert, relaxed, and responsive to your body's needs. Your success was wrapped up in your ability to stay the course. This was your job, and you achieved your goal because you did your job!

You broke your own tape. You have earned the "high five," the bow of respect from the gods of champions. Be proud, walk tall, and savor every bit of the salty taste of victory. You earned it.

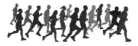

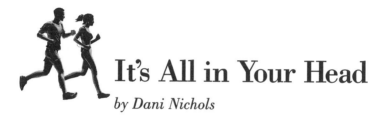

It's All in Your Head

by Dani Nichols

I have never considered myself a runner. But when I say that, I am told that running is "all in your head." To which I respond, "Then why do my legs hurt so bad?"

Running feels like a first date with that really cute, OMG guy who asks you out unexpectedly. Though I spend two weeks squealing on the phone to my gal-pals and worrying about an outfit, I'm still unprepared. I squirm and fidget, thinking I have a run in my hose and something green stuck in my teeth and why can't I ever think of anything to say? Why can't I do this?

This first date, "just a quick run" business, is no casual jog for me. I can't get my iPod earbuds to stay in—and if I manage to do so, the volume is always a bit too loud or too soft. I sweat in uncomfortable places and suddenly feel a need to itch, just when someone is looking right at me. I get very red in the face, and no matter how cute running shorts look on everybody else, they do my behind no favors. I breathe too loud, drink my water too quickly, and never know what to do when casually nodded at by a very fit, calm, and relaxed runner—other than feel a tad jealous.

I gave up running for a while but decided to start again after I got engaged. I was a couple of years out of college and had accumulated some "bored-at-a-desk-job" tummy flab. I was only a few months away from having to fit into a gorgeous white dress and being in a million pictures, so I figured that if I couldn't learn to run with that kind of motivation, when would I?

Despite that strong impetus, it still took a couple of weeks of self-talk to get me going, but one early summer evening I got home and decided to try a jog. I don't know what got into me, but I headed up the street by my apartment, ready to take on the world—or at least my street. I made it no more than a quarter of the way up the hill behind my place. One-quarter of a mile. I was defeated. I gave in to my screaming lungs and calves and walked the rest of the way. I remember resting at the top of the hill with hands on my knees, sweat in my eyes, and uncertainty in my heart. This was a much tougher resolution than I suspected, and the old ideas of "I'm not a runner" had not disappeared.

I finished my run—no, jog—no, walk—okay, stumble—in the dark that evening, and I remember looking at myself in the mirror. I was red-faced and, of course, still disappointed by my out-of-shape body and wondering if the pain was worth it. After all, billowy, fat-hiding skirts are in style these days, right?

I continued halfheartedly for another couple of months. I would get home, lace up, and head out, only to suddenly remember an urgent call I needed to make, or that my number two value meal with a large diet Coke hadn't quite settled. I'd end up just walking my route, inwardly berating myself for my lack of fortitude, unsure of how to persevere and begin to run for real.

One bright Saturday morning, my fiancé suggested that I go

running with him. He's long, lean, and built for running, and actually enjoys putting innocent feet to trail for miles. I reluctantly agreed, and we headed out to the beachside trail behind his house. True to my training, I panted for about a half-mile before giving out. "You okay?" he asked with concern. He thought when I said I'd been "running" every day that I'd actually done it—not just walked and wished I was running.

"I'm okay," I panted. "I just stink at this."

I couldn't help but feel embarrassed by my lack of athletic stamina. We didn't run together again, mostly because I didn't want to. Life got busy as the wedding approached, and I wasn't exactly eager to get back on the trail. Once we were married, my now-husband kept running and I kept pretending I was, hoping one day it would magically turn around somehow.

He kept telling me that running is all mental. "Your body can go much farther than your brain thinks it can," he insisted. But he never pressured me to go with him again, innately understanding that I needed to learn to run on my own.

One day I just got fed up. I was tired of my body, tired of making excuses for being flabby, tired of not just going and running already. So I strapped on my shoes like I always did, but this time I didn't eat first, didn't carry my cell phone, didn't even think about an iPod. I just stretched (the only two stretches I knew) and went for it, running with abandon and hoping my resolve wouldn't weaken until I was at least out of sight of the house. I was definitely panting within a half-mile but concentrated on the pier about a mile and a half away. I kept thinking about things to occupy my mind: a situation with a friend, a political discussion

I'd gotten into, a tricky situation at work. I would see a landmark ahead and think, "I'll stop when I get to that tree," but I'd arrive at the tree and suddenly see a better place farther ahead. I was panting, breathless, and tired, but my feet doggedly continued to pound the ground. I'd finally found the rhythm, one that I'd heard about so many times from other joggers but had never been able to employ myself.

Before I knew it, the pier was there, in all its seaweed-covered glory, and I was thrilled to discover that they have drinking fountains, too. I'd run farther than I had ever run before, and miraculously, I'd loved it. I was sore, breathless, and overjoyed.

Since that first run, I have learned that running is, in some ways, as much of a mental exercise as a physical one. I love early-morning jogs when the world is brand-new and dew still hangs in the air, or late-evening runs to help me process the events of my day. I'm still no marathoner, but a few months ago, I entered my first 5K and finished it. I never would have thought that possible a year ago, back when I declared myself "not a runner." My next goal is to keep up with that handsome runner-husband of mine—now that I know running really is "all in my head."

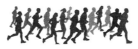

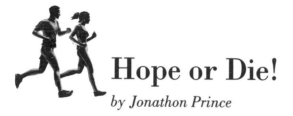

Hope or Die!

by Jonathon Prince

There I was, young and determined, running a steady pace on the shoulder of Interstate-10 across North America. All I hoped for was to get from Los Angeles, California, to Atlanta, Georgia, on foot to raise money for Hurricane Katrina victims. Had I not remained hopeful for a more comfortable twenty-five-mile run the next day, I don't know for sure that I would have been alive to see Atlanta.

I had already told everyone I knew what my plans were and what I wanted to achieve. Most of my friends and family believed my death was a certainty, that this run I planned to make was a suicide attempt at the very least. Some never leave the comfort of their hometowns; it is so much easier to settle and let life just happen. But for me to explore my imagination and to utilize my full potential, I had to do this. Something was weighing heavily on my heart and I had to see it through to the end.

That night I lie awake for hours in my sleeping bag under a clear black sky. I was completely alone, not a soul in sight for hundreds of miles; it was the heart of winter in the Texas desert and I was cold to my bones. This was nothing I wanted to get used to.

Yet it was breathtakingly beautiful, with every star appearing to be within reach. With my thoughts scattered, legs too weak to go on, and no food to replenish my body, I was in no condition to proceed alone any further. Have you ever run so far and so long that your body literally stopped working? I asked for comfort and security from whomever would listen.

Help me God, Universe, or whatever is in charge. I'm doing my part—now I need you to do yours! It's freezing cold out here! I have gone as far as I physically can and I don't want to die tonight. I need you now more then ever; please provide comfort and security and allow me to see another day.

I had been hopeless, but having no other choice, I let go of my fears, doubts, and opposing beliefs. I took a deep breath and realized I couldn't die; my reasons for living were too strong. The Universal presence acknowledged my request with a shooting star, and I accepted peace. I became calm and hopeful again, and soon I went to sleep.

Hours later, intuition woke me up just in time to notice a rat had run into my sleeping bag. Startled and wide awake from the invasion, I scared off the three growling coyotes that were creeping just yards away, looking for their morning breakfast. It clicked. *The rat was seeking comfort in my sleeping bag to keep from being eaten alive by the coyotes just yards away.* I wasn't the only one looking for hope for another day, praying for safety, comfort, and security.

That night I'd had a decision to make. I had been alone, hungry, and exhausted; I could either hope or die. My decision was simple: I chose hope. Just the hope to wake up, open my eyes, yawn, and stretch is what being so close to a frozen death had brought me to. My appreciation for life was absolute. No longer would I take the simple things in life for granted. I adopted the belief that as long as I kept on running, I'd eventually make it.

In running across the United States, I experienced a world outside of my comfort zone that I never would have realized, had I not had the courage to act on faith and follow my heart for what I believed in. Keeping my end result in mind, with a strong will, steady pulse, and a pure mind, I knew I had the tools to complete a successful run across America while helping those in need. My run did end successfully and was followed by two more runs across the country to raise money and awareness. My mission is to promote active healthy lifestyles and philanthropy by utilizing the sport of running to spread the message of hope worldwide.

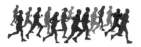

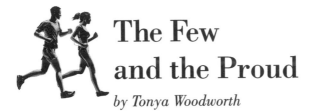

The Few
and the Proud

by Tonya Woodworth

I remember my first run-in with Master Sergeant Branch as though it was yesterday. Every bone in my body felt as though it was going to break. Given the immense pain coursing through my body, it took every ounce of willpower I had to hold back my tears. At the time, I could have sworn that death was near.

To this day, he is the most intimidating man I have ever laid my eyes on. I shudder at the mere thought of a casual run-in with him. The size of his biceps alone would be enough to intimidate even the most ruthless of criminals at San Quentin.

If he hadn't been a United States Marine, he would have been well suited for the World Wrestling Entertainment (WWE) or an Ironman competition. His build was significantly "larger" than that of an average marine; most are quite lean, thanks to constant physical activity. If you've ever met an enlisted infantryman you understand what I mean. Pinpointing just how "salty" a marine is—how high in rank and time in service—can be easily ascertained by body composition. The saltier the marine is, the less physically demanding the job usually is. The long hours of overexertion demanded of the newly enlisted causes the body to feed on muscle for energy, but when the muscles are allowed proper recovery time, the foundation is laid for a significantly stronger and more muscular build. In the case of MSgt Branch, it was clear that he had been around a while.

One of the physical requirements for a marine is physical training, or PT. At a minimum, each unit is required to implement three PT sessions per week: Mondays were usually with the platoon, Tuesdays the company, and Fridays were spent with the entire battalion. The battalion run usually consisted of a three- to five-mile run around the base at an easy pace with some calisthenics mixed in. On my first official platoon PT session, which happened to be my initial encounter with MSgt Branch, I was one of only two female marines to arrive in formation.

I wasn't alarmed to discover an abnormally high number of marines headed to sick call, although I should have been. It was a precursor for what was to come. Since the beginning of my enlistment I had been a pretty strong runner—granted, I had been competing primarily against women, but being told repeatedly that the hardest part of being a marine was getting through boot camp, I wasn't worried that day. So far, boot camp felt like a cake walk. I assured myself that I had little to be concerned about—or so I thought.

A few of the marines had come to formation hungover from a long weekend of partying. Memorial Day weekend was over, yet I could still smell the liquor lingering from the night before. I would later discover that the torture we would endure that day was more like MSgt's way of teaching the troops a lesson in self-control. He despised those who came to formation hungover and felt, I suspect, that it was an obvious act of disrespect, not only to him, but to the Marine Corps as well.

Much to my surprise, the run began at a fairly rapid pace. I am barely five feet tall; each one of my strides was just half of that of the men's. I had to double up my pace just to stay in the game. It wasn't long before I began to lag behind. No matter how hard I pushed myself, I just couldn't keep up. My eyes began to burn profusely as the sweat poured off my body. Every inch of me began to ache. I felt as though my chest would cave in at any moment. I was in a full-out sprint for the first mile, but no matter how hard I pushed myself, neither my lungs nor my legs could keep up. I gradually lost sight of the platoon. And because "you never leave a marine behind," MSgt Branch halted the troops and made them "drop and give him twenty"—twenty push-ups, twenty flutter-kicks, twenty crunches—you name it, they did it. A sense of relief washed over me as I drew closer to them. My lungs hurt so badly, and for a brief second I was hopeful of finally catching a breather. Calisthenics were the easiest exercise for me. It was a task that I had no problem outperforming the men in—a feat I am most proud of. Unfortunately, as soon as I caught up with them, MSgt Branch had the troops up and running again. This cat-and-mouse game went on for nearly ten miles, although I didn't know the distance at the time. If I had, I would have given up for sure. Not knowing proved to be a blessing in disguise.

The run itself was grueling. At times it made me feel weak and unsure of myself and my abilities as a marine. Listening to any man of MSgt Branch's caliber berate you and tell you that the effort you were putting forth wasn't good enough would appear to be counterproductive in the eyes of most. However, after all was said and done and we were back in formation and standing in the parking lot outside our shop, this man I had begun to loathe stood in front of the formation and congratulated us. We proved, not only to him, but to ourselves, that we had the ability to persevere—a true testament to the Marine Corps and to ourselves. This was a task that most would have given up on, he exclaimed. Once the pain started to kick in, many civilians would have quit and walked away, or just as those who had gone to sick call that day, they would have been defeated by fear from the start and never would have attempted the task at all. This is what made us unique. This is what made us worthy of being "The Few. The Proud." My heart filled with pride, both to be a marine and to have overcome my own pain to continue the run.

If I could take any lesson from that day, it would be that there will always be challenges in our lives. It is how we overcome these challenges and the knowledge that we gain from them that are most important. We don't always know how we will get to our destination in life, but we cannot be immobilized by fear. We must have faith and believe in ourselves and let that be our guide. Thank you, MSgt Branch, for this life lesson. I am forever in your debt.

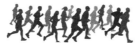

Going the Extra Mile(s) When You're Running on Empty

by Pat Williams

"The world expects results. Don't tell others
about the pain. Show them the baby!"

—Jeff Galloway

I have acquired a rather sadistic hobby for one who long ago surpassed middle-age: I run marathons. Actually, some wouldn't call it running. It is more like a diligent, spirited walk. Realizing that misery not only loves company but often insists on it, and being the heady salesman that I am, I convinced my wife, Ruth, to run them with me. So in 1997, ten days after our wedding, we ran the Boston Marathon together. At the nine-mile mark, Ruth pulled up, told me her knee was hurt, and that she had to stop at a first-aid station. Her parting words were: "Keep going. Don't quit. I love you."

I pushed onward. For eleven miles, I shuttled along by myself with thoughts of a sidelined Ruth troubling my weary head. *How disappointed she must be! I hope she doesn't feel that she let me down.* It was at the twenty-mile mark that I wheezed up Boston's Heartbreak Hill, my strength waning, my legs cramping, and my heart pounding. I thought I was about to hit the proverbial wall.

Then I heard a voice. "Paaatrick!" Was someone calling my name?

Then I heard it again, louder this time. "Paaaatrick!" I peered over my right shoulder and thought I was hallucinating. But I wasn't. There she was, running toward me in her canary yellow shirt. She was waving at me with a huge smile on her face.

Her knee had been treated and she had run eleven miles to catch up to me. We ran the last six miles together. At the last mile marker—mile twenty-six—Ruth stopped for a moment to put on her lipstick before we turned the final corner. You know the saying, "It ain't over 'til the fat lady sings." Well, for Ruth, it ain't over 'til the lipstick goes on. As we turned on to Boylston Street, we held hands and ran that last quarter-mile to the finish line.

There are two didactic "legs" to this story. The first is that I might be the slowest marathon runner in the history of the Boston Marathon. But we'll concern ourselves with that at another time. The second is that perseverance is paramount. Nothing is accomplished by quitting before reaching the finish line of any undertaking, by caving to challenges. Ruth did not give up on finding me or finishing the marathon with me.

I tell this story illustrating the reality of marathoning because it is the most vivid example I can summon concerning one's ability to push ahead amid the daunting collar of perceived or real limitations. Marathons reflect life. You get to practice "not quitting" for about five hours.

I learned that Ruth won't quit when life gets hard or you have setbacks and heartaches. Through twelve years of marriage— through raising children—Ruth remains as tenacious today as she was that day at the Boston Marathon, running determinedly in her canary yellow shirt.

Japanese psychiatrist Shoma Morita encapsulated a marathoner's stick-to-itiveness when he wrote, "When running up a hill, it is all right to give up as many times as you wish as long as your feet keep moving."

That's good advice for us all!

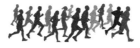

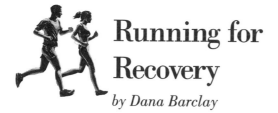

Running for Recovery

by Dana Barclay

I stared up at the treadmill, feeling weak and dispirited. Beyond dispirited, actually—more like the spirit had been cut out of me over the past thirty days in alcohol rehab, which I'd euphuistically dubbed "winter camp." I'd been home for a month, and life without alcohol wore at me like a hair shirt. I was very unhealthy and out of touch, not only with my mind and body, but with myself. There was nothing to fill the void that alcohol left. Alcohol had been one of my best friends for many years. Losing that friend left me in mourning; sad and distraught. Yet a little voice inside me said get up off the floor and walk. So I got up, got on the treadmill, and began to walk.

I walked again the following day, and the day after that. Eventually, I mounted a television/video player to watch while I walked. Gradually, I realized I felt better. That's when I started running. The first quarter mile almost killed me, but I did it again the next day and it became easier. The *Band of Brothers* series and all seven seasons of *The West Wing* accompanied my progress to running a twelve-minute mile. I felt triumphant and powerful afterward, as if I had scaled a huge mountain or some other magnificent feat.

I was getting back in touch with my body and that felt extraordinary. I didn't run to lose weight. It wasn't a vanity thing. Well, it was a vanity of sorts. I needed to feel better about myself, know that I could do something, and be something, besides a drinker. And running helped. I felt less stress and worry and felt better physically than I had in a long time.

I started a running log book as I began to run faster and farther. I purchased good running shoes and socks. I also researched other components of a runner's lifestyle—food, vitamins, stretches—and found inspiration from various running gurus and their articles and tips. I realized that I wasn't just running—I was building a brand new lifestyle for myself. And I thought, *Cool!* Running was becoming an essential element of my new life.

At four hundred miles I replaced my running shoes.

It wasn't until I began to run trails outside that running transitioned from a lifestyle to a spiritual experience. I felt connected to the world and at peace with it when I ran, as I did at no other time. It was meditative, a time when I relaxed and drifted in an almost out-of-body, runner's-high state. I learned to sort out the stresses of the day and leave problems behind, trailing and falling behind me like the wake following a boat. I had connected with my mind, body, and spirit in ways I had never experienced previously. Feelings of powerlessness and low self-esteem were replaced with empowerment and confidence. My once-unbalanced life now had focus, balance, and self-control.

I have been lucky enough to run in some inspiring places: steamy sunrise beach runs in the Caribbean, and cool, quiet, wooded trails up north. Others have been perhaps not as inspiring, yet fruitful: on hotel treadmills and busy city streets. I work running into my life no matter where life takes me.

Running changed again after I was talked into running in my first 5K race. I remember being so nervous as the start approached, I thought I was going to be sick. My goal was just to finish without walking—I did, and I was hooked. I did well for my age group, placing well above runners much younger than myself. I have been racing ever since.

My greatest triumph was just recently when I won the grand masters trophy in a local 8K race. I was the fastest female over fifty years of age and got a PR (personal record) too. I have come a very long way since that day I was sitting on the basement floor, staring up at the treadmill and feeling so terribly broken and lost.

Running has become a tool for self-discovery and has taught me how to deal, not only with addiction, but with life's problems, stresses, and joys. Prior to becoming a runner, my addiction fed my self-destructive attitudes and habits. Running assisted me, one step at a time, to overcome these habits. Running helped me find balance, and the focus that helps me feel increasingly confident and in control, rather than powerless, weak, and victimized. Instead, I feel in harmony with my mind, body, and spirit. I believe this has happened for me through running.

And most important, I don't miss drinking.

The Other End of the Day: Ironman USA

by Megan Williams

Probably at no other time in my life will I have a woman my grandmother's age extend an arm that's the texture of a baked potato and offer me Vaseline to put between my legs.

Nor will I see adult men and women licking their armpits.

Nor hear a fifty-year-old man exclaim proudly, "I think I'm gonna be much faster now that I've shaved my pubic area."

This is the world of the long-distance triathlon—like all the worlds we construct, both fictional and nonfictional, it has a way of wrapping us up. It comes to seem so completely natural that when I complain to a friend that I faded to run 3:23 in the last six miles of the Boston Marathon, he suggests I start doing thirty-mile runs. So what if this means running from Philadelphia to Trenton? He's done Hawaii three times—he should know.

I have a background in ballet, gymnastics, and equestrian events, but triathlon is the most ritualized sport I've ever participated in. I've seen a man spend thousands of dollars on aerodynamic wheels and aerobars for his bike, all to shave off a couple of precious seconds—and then ride the Ironman course with a giant stuffed animal between his handle bars for good luck.

For eight weekends before Ironman Lake Placid, I'm on my bike at 6:00 AM, facing a 100-mile ride and then an hour run. To say that the Ironman training is consuming would be an understatement. When you are running more than 50 miles a week, biking more than 200 miles, and swimming more than 4 miles, you don't have time for much else. A married friend of mine whose husband does long-distance triathlons fondly refers to Ironman USA as Lake Flaccid; many spouses and significant others complain that they are no longer "allowed" to do Ironman because of the time the training requires. At the Ironman expo before the race, almost every imaginable product is for sale with the M-Dot (Ironman) label on it—except Ironman condoms. The race itself is the best form of birth control. What could possibly make you feel less "in the mood" than inner-thigh chaffing or the night sweats that come with overtraining?

While ballet dancers chew beeswax for the empty calories, my friends and I can, and do, spend hours discussing what to wear and eat on our 100-mile bike rides. If we are going to be in the saddle for six-plus hours, we need to be comfortable and eat the proper food. Something about all this planning allows us to rationalize and control the undeniable fact that no matter what precautions we take, we are going to be miserable at some point during the nine to thirteen hours it takes to complete this triathlon.

When friends of mine ask if they can watch me run, I tell them no. This race can get ugly. Why would I want people around with cameras if chances are good that I will shit or throw up all over myself?

If you had told me six years ago that I would be treading water at the start line of Ironman Lake Placid with 1,800 other people, I would have laughed. And probably lit up another cigarette. At that point in my life, as a first-year Ph.D. student in English, running a marathon and doing a triathlon lay within my vague conception of myself, but not within its reality. I looked like any other graduate student of English—dressed mostly in black and decorated with numerous piercings. I smoked a pack a day and had that pasty complexion that comes from being able to talk convincingly about lesbian writers from the Caribbean diaspora. In 1996, how was I to know that a plan to quit smoking would lead me into ten marathons and to the start line of a race that included a 2.4-mile ocean swim, 112-mile bike ride, and 26.2-mile run?

On the beach of Mirror Lake in Lake Placid, I am surrounded by people spraying themselves with PAM cooking spray to slip more easily into their wetsuits.

"Want some?" Margaret offers.

"Yuck. I feel enough like a human sausage as it is."

"At least it's not like that ocean swim in New Jersey where we all looked like shark bait in our seal-colored wetsuits."

I laugh and am surprised. My whole life I have been afraid of the things I could not do, but for some reason I am not afraid of this race.

Margaret hikes her bathing-suit bottoms up into a giant wedgie and asks a neighbor to put BODYGLIDE on her butt cheeks. She grins at me over her shoulder. "No dignity in triathlon."

I thought that the week before Ironman would be like the days before my first marathon, the Pittsburgh Marathon. On the way there I'd been stricken by a panic attack so severe that I left clammy spots on the steering wheel and seat of my rental car.

"I-snuffle-snuffle-CAN'T-sob-DO-sniffle-THIS," I stuttered over the phone to my boyfriend. The pressure and doubt that I would not be able to run 26.2 miles the next morning were so strong that I felt as if a fist were pressing against my chest. I would hate myself if I couldn't finish the marathon, but I would hate myself more for not even starting it. Either way, I hated myself for this fear and self-doubt. My boyfriend talked me out of my panic, and I finished my first marathon in a semi-respectable 3:52.

Even so, the old self-doubt remained, and no amount of running seemed to make it disappear.

But during the week leading up to Lake Placid, I'm curiously calm. Maybe I've moved beyond self-doubt, or maybe the distances in this race are so huge that I can't wrap my mind around them. I read article after article in an effort to discover what the experience of racing in this event will be like. One thing all the writers agree on: I will go through a hundred different emotions and extremes during the course of the day.

Like Frederick the mouse in the children's story who stores up colors and images for the long winter ahead, as part of my prerace strategy I start to stockpile images. In those inevitable moments of self-doubt, I will think of all the people in my life who have told me that I wouldn't be able to do something: the woman who tutored me when I was ten and said I might not ever be able to learn to read well, my high school cross-country coach who discounted me as a pseudo-athlete. I will remember that my university did not reappoint me this fall, that I have osteoporosis and some freak pulmonary disease called sarcoidosis. Pure fury will propel me across the finish line.

But not once during the race do I think of these things. When the cannon explodes at 7:00 AM and the largest wave-start in triathlon history splashes off, all heading for the same buoy, I am thinking about how quiet swimming is. Above water you hear the buzz of splashing and kicking, but below you feel a primordial darkness. I can't see the bottom of Mirror Lake, but I can see the bubbles from the scuba divers lurking beneath. I think they are there to videotape us. Later, I learn that their real job is to push the swimmers up who get caught under the blanket of bodies and can't find their way back to the surface.

Triathlon has strict rules to keep its competitors from talking to one another. The silence of the swim is a given, but on the bike we must maintain three bike-lengths distance from each other to avoid drafting. By the time the run comes and you're allowed to talk to each other, you are too tired. Gone are the camaraderie and the companionship that you find on 100-mile training rides with your friends.

In Ironman competition, you have to do it alone and in silence.

The night before the race I go to an Episcopal blessing of the athletes, mostly to keep Margaret company. Leave it to the Episcopalians to devise an Iron blessing; a Catholic service would have made us feel guilty for devoting so much time to our minds and bodies. But something the minister says stays in my mind during the twelve hours, nineteen minutes, and fifteen seconds it takes to get me to the finish line. "No matter how you do, whether you finish or not, something about this event will change you forever."

This blessing reminds me that I have had my share of mornings when I wondered how I was going to summon the energy to make myself a cup of coffee, much less make it through a whole day of coaching and teaching. After breaking up with a boyfriend or living through my parents' divorce, I have stood in the winter air and waited next to the train tracks in North Philadelphia. At those times, breathing in the diesel and creosote that accompanied my daily commute, I thought about jumping, but something always stopped me. This something, this fight when you are at rock bottom, this absolute refusal to be overtaken by the bleakness of a March day, is what I feel most at Ironman.

I am amazed not so much by my own ability to endure, as by the energy that surrounds me. I don't feel in awe of myself for finally "completing the dream." I don't feel exultation at the finish line when the announcer shouts for the 777th time that day, "You are an Ironman." What I feel at every stage—as I follow people out of the water and hobble after them to our bikes—is amazement that we are all doing this. They carry me through the race, not by their words, but by their actions. There is a picture of me at the beginning of the run with a huge scowl on my face. Clearly, I'm thinking about the 26.2 miles still ahead. But I know that I wouldn't have had the courage to start if I were not following someone else.

People ask me if the race hurt, and I answer "of course." Of course it hurt, but unlike the rest of life, it is a hurt that you can plan. Sure, I cursed my way through a large part of the bike-ride portion. And contrary to the rest of my competitors, I didn't think the scenery was particularly spectacular. During the last ten miles of the fifty-six-mile bike loop that you do twice, you climb 2,000 feet up the side of Whiteface Mountain. Sure, it's beautiful. Huge outcroppings tower over the road and "falling rock" signs are everywhere. But all I'm thinking on the second loop is, *Why does this have to be so difficult?* Then I remember that this is something I have chosen to do, and that keeps me pedaling. And finally I am at the top of the last series of hills, called Mama Bear, Papa Bear, and Baby Bear.

"Do I look like friggin' Goldilocks?" I shout out of pure joy to the spectators at the top of the hill.

"What you look like is way too perky," an old man screams after me. I giggle and keep riding toward transition.

Mostly, what I feel during the race is this amazing awe at the endurance of the human spirit. I am soundly beaten by several men over fifty, and coming up a hill on the run course, I pass a man doing the whole race in a wheelchair. This is his third time trying to finish, and this time he does.

My most memorable moments in the race occur on the run course. There are 3,000 permanent residents in Lake Placid, and over 3,000 race volunteers. To the runners, it feels as if each and every one comes out to cheer. Each mile marker is its own city, filled with people offering sponges for your face, chicken broth for the salt content, fruit, cookies, Gatorade, GU Energy products, you name it. At every aid station, people shout encouragement to walkers and runners alike.

"What can I get you? What can I get you?" a ten-year-old boy yells at mile thirteen.

"Um, new legs?"

He laughs, and I keep running. "You guys are so awesome," he shouts to my back.

As the finish line inches closer, I begin to wonder what's so awesome about devoting twenty or more hours a week to your training? To yourself? Surely triathlon must be the most solipsistic and narcissistic sport in the world. It's certainly one of the few sports where I can date men who shave more of their bodies than I do. We devote hours and hours to our bodies and our minds. We probably listen more to our heart-rate monitors than we do to our loved ones. Triathletes, myself included, are some of the most selfish and self-involved people I have ever met. But ultimately, as I spend the last miles of Ironman Lake Placid thinking about that pudgy ten-year-old's "awesome" comment, I realize that this focus is the very thing that saves us.

At the last mile marker, a woman on crutches hands me a slice of orange. I thank her, and she turns to face me.

"No, thank *you*. Thank all of you guys. You are awesome. An inspiration."

And there it is again. The final confirmation that Ironman is not so much a testimony to one's individual strength as it is a testimony to the universal human spirit to endure in all its ugliness and beauty.

"Yes. Ironman was difficult," I tell the people who are interested enough to ask. "But I would recommend it to anyone." As often as not, these people laugh and tell me I'm crazy. Maybe I am, and maybe a 140.6-mile race is a long way to go to eradicate self-doubt. But if you are like me, and are afraid of so many things, maybe Ironman will become one of those images that you can save in case you ever again feel that life has hit you with something that you are not strong enough to fight.

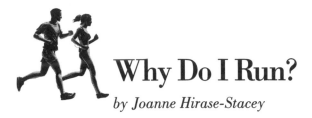

Why Do I Run?

by Joanne Hirase-Stacey

People often ask me why I run. My standard response has always been, "So I can eat anything I want." But lately, I've given my running habit more thought . . . especially when my knees and feet hurt, when it's too cold or too hot, or when my list of tasks is so long I know I need thirty hours in the day to accomplish everything.

So I reached deep into my soul while pounding my soles on the road. What I discovered is there isn't just one reason I lace up my shoes every day. Running is my lifelong companion. One I can depend on any time, any place.

Running is about getting to the heart of the matter. The body, no matter what shape or size, is remarkable. I feel most alive when my blood is flowing through my veins, my arms are pumping, and my legs are propelling me forward. The little aches and pains I experience are mere reminders of what I accomplish step by step.

And step by step I keep pace with myself. Running is my time. No phone, no Internet, no television. No to-do list, no meetings, no interruptions. It's my personal sanity check. When everything is hectic and noisy, I collapse into my running self, and the only sounds I hear are my rhythmic breathing and my footfalls. I challenge myself by pushing hard, or I take control by running at a nice steady tempo, or I empower myself by running any way I feel.

Sometimes my impulse is to run and get away from my problems. When I put distance between myself and whatever is amiss in my world, my troubles evaporate for a brief time. Sometimes I even manage to solve dilemmas that seem overwhelming. Running clears my mind; my thoughts are peaceful. And when I think I can't do something, then figure out it's not impossible, my attitude changes. It's the same feeling as when I crest that daunting hill and think I'm on top of the world, absolutely invincible.

So invincible, I am my own superhero. When I'm running, I'm unstoppable: I soar, I bound, I leap. There is no running goal I can't achieve, whether it's finishing a half marathon, running a fast 10K, or just getting out the door. My neighbors think I'm crazy when they drive by and see me running through the snow, in the rain, or in the heat of the day. But they haven't seen me in a cape or with a golden lasso yet, so they don't know about my secret action-hero life!

Luckily, my battles are small and I'm free to walk outside my door and go. I don't have to worry about car bombs or missiles. I'm not debilitated by cancer or leukemia or any other illness or disease. I have two arms, two legs, ten fingers, ten toes. I'm not bedridden or in a wheelchair. Or dead. The only thing I have to fight is myself when I come up with excuses and don't feel like moving. I run for my mom, whose dementia is getting worse by the day. I run for my dad, who is unsteady on his feet. I run for my aunts, for my uncles, for my cousins, for my friends, and even for people I don't know who face serious issues in their daily lives. Each mile I log is a testament to myself, and a celebration of my being. It's one way to show the world who I am.

In my quest for a better answer of why I run, I'm amazed at the numerous reasons I come up with. But to keep it simple I now say, "I run because I can."

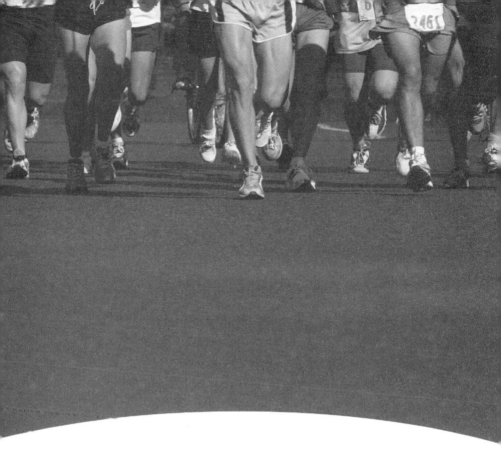

The Social Side
of the Sneakers

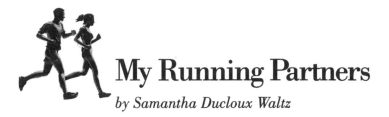

My Running Partners

by Samantha Ducloux Waltz

"Want to start running with me?" I asked my neighbor as I pushed a caramel mocha across her kitchen table to sweeten the deal.

"And why would I want to do this?" Sheri eyed me suspiciously.

"Fitness. Serenity. A runner's high." Articles in a running magazine I'd been given had me so enthusiastic that I'd already bought running shoes.

Sheri sipped her mocha. "Nice promises. We'll have to go early."

We agreed on 5:45 AM—a ghastly hour—so our husbands would be with our still-sleeping children. We'd be back to get families off to work and school.

I immediately fell in love with running. That morning, I shut off the alarm at the first buzz, pulled on a shirt, shorts, and my new running shoes, and slipped out the door into the crisp autumn air. As I jogged the block to Sheri's, the sun crept up the eastern sky. It illuminated Mt. Hood, an hour's drive away, with streaks of pale orange and soft pink. Somewhere a dog yipped, and lights blinked on in houses along our route as our neighborhood awakened to a new day.

Sheri shared my enthusiasm. Blocks grew to miles over the first two months as we ran the hills of our neighborhood and traded the deepest secrets of our hearts, marveling at our weight loss and energy boost.

Each morning I hummed as I fed my golden retriever, Rex, and my cat, Snooper, then woke Hal with a kiss and tousled each of my three children's hair as I got them up. Everyone benefited from my high spirits.

Fall faded into winter. Darkness lengthened, the air turned cold, and rain often pelted our hooded jackets. "This isn't fun any more," Sheri announced one day as we headed out.

I spent every inch of our three-mile run coaxing her to keep running.

"Winters are for hibernation," she insisted. No quantity of caramel mochas could change her mind.

Hal insisted I get a safety vest, wristband ID, and pepper spray. A lime-green jacket with wide, reflective stripes over my clothing, a wrist band strapped on my wrist, and pepper spray zipped into my fanny pack, I hit the road alone. I missed Sheri, but for several days my runs felt glorious. My arms and legs were pistons; my mind was clear and sharp. But after a few weeks I started feeling a bit lonely and very vulnerable. I needed a new running partner.

"Want to run with me?" I asked Rex as I poured a cup of kibbles in his bowl.

"He'd never bite anybody," Hal grumbled. "Lick them to death, maybe."

"Whoever sees an eighty pound dog at my side will leave me alone."

"I hope so," he said.

I kissed his cheek. "I'll be fine," I promised. I didn't like worrying him, but I couldn't give up running.

"Heel," I commanded Rex on our first morning running together.

But I hadn't trained him to heel very well, and I'd never taught him to start slow and build up to a comfortable, steady pace. *Sprint, yank, sprint, yank* was our pace as we sputtered up the road.

"Heel," I ordered again, more firmly this time. Now Rex was too busy examining shrubs for interesting scents, and leaving his own scent behind, to pay me any attention.

"Heel," I insisted when we met another dog on the road, but Rex had to circle his new friend, nose to tail, before we went on. Twice I nearly fell when he tangled the leash around my feet as he darted after a squirrel.

I worked with him for a week before I gave up. "He didn't cut it," I whined to Hal. "I wish you could run with me." But we both knew he couldn't leave the kids.

Once again I headed out by myself. I was relieved that there was no leash to pull at my shoulder or trip me up, and I ran easily for the first mile. Then the dark closed in around me. Something rustled in the bushes on my left and my stomach clenched. I thought of Sheri, snuggled in her bed, as I trotted home. Maybe I should just snuggle in my own bed; 5:45 AM was a ridiculous time to get up anyway.

"Meow." Snooper, our cat, padded over to me as I slipped in the front door, and rubbed against my leg.

"Hi, kitty." I lifted her in my arms and she licked my cheek with her sandpaper tongue.

"I had a lousy run," I told her, stroking her silky gray fur. "I wish you weighed another hundred pounds. I need someone to run with me."

A gravelly purr started deep in her throat. She sounded a lot happier than I felt.

The next morning I had to talk firmly with myself as I tied on my running shoes. It wasn't the rain. I was used to that. I'd even jogged in snow, more dependent on my morning run than on a cup of coffee. The days were lengthening now and I had a bit of predawn light. It was the creepy noises, the yards of near-darkness between the street lamps, the sense of being entirely alone if anything should happen to me that unsettled me.

Crack. A branch snapped beside me. My chest tightened and I broke rhythm. *Steady*, I told myself. Any scurrying creature could do that. I ran on. More rustling in the shrubs of the next yard. Was someone stalking me?

These are normal morning sounds, I reassured myself, resisting the temptation to dash home.

In the next yard I noticed a lean, gray body loping across a broad swatch of lawn. An opossum? They didn't run that fast. A raccoon? They were slower, too. It was hard to tell in the near-darkness. Maybe just a cat.

The creature darted into the rhododendrons lining the side yard of the next house, then shot across the lawn. It was a cat. I'd have sworn it was Snooper, but I was more than a mile from home.

Several blocks farther on I sighted the cat again. This time a street lamp flooded the yard.

"Snooper. That is you," I cried.

He darted back into a hedge of azaleas. Apparently he wanted his presence to be a secret.

I laughed. My spirits lifted and my stride lengthened. I wasn't sure what good my self-appointed bodyguard could do. If I twisted my ankle would he race home and yowl until someone followed him and found me? But I appreciated his effort.

I was still smiling when a snarling German shepherd leapt off a porch and bounded toward me, barking ferociously. It would be at my throat before I could retrieve my pepper spray. When the German shepherd was less than ten yards from me, a hissing ball of fur hurled itself at the dog's throat. Diverted from its original goal, the shepherd slid to a stop, lowered its head, and growled at Snooper.

Snooper wasn't much bigger than the dog's head, but he stopped just yards from it, back arched, hair bristling.

I had my pepper spray now but didn't want to spray my cat. If I jumped between them, I'd be torn to pieces. Waves of terror washed over me. I was about to watch my beloved cat be eaten alive.

Snooper hissed and spit, ignoring the dog's warning growls. He was fifteen pounds of pure rage. The shepherd backed up. Snooper kept up his full-court press. The shepherd backed up another step. Then it whirled on its haunches and raced back to the porch, Snooper nipping at its heels.

Back on the porch, the dog continued to bark menacingly, but Snooper just glared at it with his unblinking yellow eyes, then turned away, as if to say, *Come on. Is that the best you can do?*

"Hey, thanks." I reached down to swoop my brave rescuer into my arms.

Usually an affectionate cat, he dodged me and proceeded sedately to the next yard where he waited for me to start running again. He was on duty. I could thank him later.

"A feline running partner, eh?" Hal said when I recounted our adventure. "I'd still keep the pepper spray."

I'd do that, but I doubted I'd need it with Snooper at my side. I should go shopping right away for a catnip mouse. He'd like that a lot better than a caramel mocha.

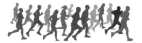

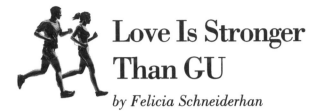

Love Is Stronger Than GU

by Felicia Schneiderhan

I ran my third marathon six days before our wedding.

At the Saturday expo, I was picking up my number when I turned around to see Mark whipping out his checkbook. He had run four marathons before, but he was in no shape to do one now. Not only did he not have the training, he didn't have the gear—he was wearing shoes that had seen two marathons. But the hype of the premarathon expo snagged him; he signed up and bought some shorts and enough GU Energy Gel to last him the 26.2 miles he had not trained for.

We were in love, we were getting married, and we were running a marathon together!

The morning of the Quad Cities Marathon was overcast and cool. Mark and I crossed the Interstate-74 Bridge over the Mississippi River, traipsed around Bettendorf, Iowa, and skipped along the river into Davenport. Around mile ten we crossed back into Illinois via the Centennial Bridge, and it was here that Mark fell behind. I waited for him at the foot of the bridge, but it looked like the air had seeped out of his tires.

"The arches in my shoes are flat," he said. "I know you love me and I love you, but we don't have to stay together."

I knew I couldn't run at his slower pace, so I left my fiancé at the bridge.

Three more easy miles and I ascended another bridge to Arsenal Island. I was halfway there. But because I was with the slower runners, all the fans were gone. With no friendly faces in sight my spirits sank. That's when the head trip started. I felt a pain in my right IT (iliotibial) band, shooting up and down my leg. Mile fourteen, mile fifteen—*Just keep going*, I told myself. *Run it because you can, because you won't have to do this ever again.* Mile sixteen, mile seventeen. I came upon three people sitting in lawn chairs, their boom box blasting a commercial. *Just make it to mile eighteen. At eighteen you'll be off the island—you can quit then.* I reached the aid station and took a cup of Gatorade from a hand.

"Good job, Felicia!" I looked up to see Christine smiling at me. She'd been my friend in junior high, and I hadn't seen her for more than a decade. "Keep going!" she cheered. I found the strength to pick it up for another mile. I knew my parents would be waiting at mile twenty. *Just make it to twenty and then you can quit—no shame in going twenty.* At mile twenty Mom and Dad cheered, "Keep going! Keep going!" I dug down deep and kept going.

The last six miles included a hairpin turn at mile twenty-three. I could see people in front looping back around toward me as they made their way to the finish line. We cheered each other on. As I continued around the sharp turn and geared up for those last three miles, I knew there would be no more friendly faces. I was going to have to do this alone.

And then, in the distance, heading toward me at the beginning of the hairpin turn, his insoles shot, his arches flat, I saw Mark—still running.

"SCHNEIDERHAN!" I yelled.

Mark was at mile twenty-two; I was at twenty-four. I grabbed him and pulled him into my lane (so technically he skipped two miles, but who cares?). We talked about all we had seen along the race, and before I knew it, we crossed the finish line. The race was so small they announced both our names. The clock said 5:01.

You can train like an Olympian and spend thousands on gear and only eat organic for months, but when it comes down to race day, you'll never make it without the love.

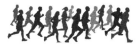

Those Who Can, Run, and Those Who Can't . . .

by Kim Dent Karrick

School was finally out for the summer. It would be one of the hottest summers on record. A lot of records would be broken over the next couple of months; the Summer Olympics were in full swing with Bruce Jenner making America proud and inspiring young athletes of all abilities. I was twelve years old, and that summer my feet grew an entire size! That certainly wasn't that big of a deal; it didn't make the evening news. But it did mean a new pair of tennis shoes immediately, instead of just prior to the start of school in the fall, as was the usual routine at our house.

A fabulous pair of red, white, and blue Zips were my shoes of choice—I'm telling you, they looked fast just sitting in their shoebox. I felt so inspired looking at them. I put them on and was ready to race; I was going to set a record. I handed our bright blue Big Ben alarm clock to my younger sister and I headed for the street. My sister watched the second hand come around to twelve and then screamed, "On your mark, get set, go!" I shot out like a sprayed cockroach, pretty sure smoke was coming out from my heels.

I made it about a quarter of a mile before I collapsed on the curb, grabbing my legs and yelling in pain. When my sister finally strolled down, I told her to go get Mom and Dad to rescue me with the car. I was sure I'd broken both my legs. This was my introduction to shin splints and the beginning of many years of being the butt of family jokes.

It was also the end of my running career. Sure, I've run/walked the Crescent City Classic in New Orleans with family and friends a few times, and participated in the End-to-End Walk in Bermuda (26.2 miles). But that's been enough for me.

I have, however, spent countless hours and weekends since then cheering on my dad and sister at numerous 5K, 10K, and even half marathons. These days, I cheer my husband on at everything from 5Ks to duathlons to Ironman triathlon competitions. I've bandaged toes, run (not far) for cold towels, pumped bike tires, made peanut butter and jelly sandwiches and thermoses of hot chicken soup for my husband to grab as he passes by during his all-day races. I've stayed up all night for fear the alarm clock wouldn't go off and my husband's months of training would go down the tubes if we overslept. I've been cold enough to turn blue, stood too long in the sun and turned red, just to catch a two-second glimpse of my racer on the course and yell his name. I've pushed the bike back to the hotel, carried gear bags as big as I am, and I still cry every time my pale, sweaty, and always-smiling husband crosses the finish line.

Sometimes, I get caught up in all of the excitement at those races and I think to myself, *maybe I'll train and do this race next year.* Then, I close my eyes so I can see myself crossing the finish line . . . but all I see are those patriotic-looking Zips and me lying on the curb!

Four-Legged Running Partners

by Joanne Hirase-Stacey

My running partners have four legs. Maggie, my Belgian shepherd, isn't as fond of running as Isamu, my rottweiler, but she always wants to go just to see what's happening in the world outside our home. It's quite the daily ritual—they see my running shoes go on and they sit by the back door and cry. If I take too long, they'll charge into the bedroom to find me and make sure I'm still going.

Putting a harness on an eager dog isn't easy. Usually my husband, Bill, will get the dogs "dressed" while I'm getting ready. Isamu jumps up and down and twirls around and wiggles and squirms. Maggie is good. She sits and waits until she hears the snap of the clasp before she starts pacing. They each have their own way of warming up.

I only take one dog at a time. I'd prefer to take Maggie first because she's slower and would be a nice way for me to ease into my run. But Isamu goes first because he's full of energy, and he will break things or leave little accidents all over the place if he's left behind. I once tried running with both of them at the same time, but they were too strong and my arms hurt for a few days after. Not to mention the fact they each tried to go in a different direction and discovered my arms don't stretch.

I don't take them out in the winter (falling on the ice is only fun when you're ice skating). I did see a treadmill for dogs, but Bill refuses to let me buy one. So every spring I have to reteach them the concept of pacing. Because they are so enthusiastic, they bolt out the door, dragging me behind, only to stop a half mile later, tired and out of breath. I try to keep the leash short, but it isn't always effective because it cuts off the circulation in my hand when they pull. But it only takes a week or so for them to remember they have to start slower to go longer.

We live on a mountain pass, so there are dirt roads and hills galore, perfect for running. And we see interesting critters along the way. Sometimes deer leap out at us, silent and graceful. White rabbits scamper across the road to hide in the brush, then follow us with their little eyes as we pass. We've had pheasants squawk and dive-bomb us before they glide back up into the endless sky. We even heard a mountain lion scream—we probably got too close to her babies for her liking. Sometimes there are cattle on the road that think we're trying to herd them, so they trot along slowly ahead of us dropping cow pies along the way. The horses grazing in the pastures perk up their ears to see what we're doing. And the coyotes watch us from up high, occasionally yipping to catch our attention. These distractions and the beautiful scenery always make our runs exciting and enjoyable.

Last year, Maggie and Isamu helped me train for a half marathon, so I shared my finisher's medal and third-place trophy with them. They were excited because I was excited, but their interest waned once they discovered I didn't have an edible prize.

We just added a third dog to the pack, a pit bull named Zebekiah. Now that I have three running partners, I decided to change my training strategy. I'll take Isamu for distance, Zebekiah for speed work, and Maggie, well, she'll just go for fun. You never know, maybe with this new training regimen I can turn a third-place win into second or even first.

The greatest thing about having live-in running partners is they get me out the door and force me to run. I can't look into those big brown eyes and deny them their time out in the world without feeling guilty. I don't want to disappoint them, so no matter my mood or my schedule, we run.

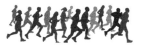

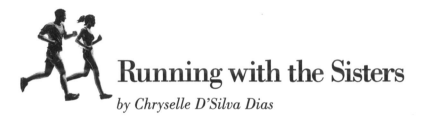

Running with the Sisters

by Chryselle D'Silva Dias

I t was the unusual, quirky name that first caught my eye.

Left on a table in my town's library was a small blue leaflet advertising a local running group for women called "Running Sisters." The cartoon logo showed three women running, arms akimbo and hair flying. I loved the name, and the logo made me laugh.

It had only been a few months since I had been in England, having moved from India earlier that year after my marriage to an Indian doctor practicing in the U.K. I had no family or friends in this new, cold country, and the library was starting to be a good place to spend my time.

Running was never part of my plans. My sporting activity was limited to dismal performances in 100-meter races in school and the occasional throw-ball and cricket games with the neighborhood children. In 2004, as a volunteer with the Samaritans Helpline (a suicide prevention service in Mumbai), I put together a fund-raising and publicity effort for Samaritans as part of the first-ever Mumbai Marathon. A team of us ran the "Dream Run" along with thousands of other novice runners and celebrities.

Practicing for that run wasn't easy, though. Indian women don't run—not on the streets, anyway. And certainly not for the sheer fun of it. For a girl growing up in urban India, running is fraught with perils worse than stopwatches. The lack of pavement or designated sport areas means braving the dusty roads full of streaming traffic, even at 6:00 AM. Then, there are the men. Men behind the wheels of public-transport buses, trucks, cars, motorcycles, even bicycles—all of whom thrive on intimidating a woman who is running alone.

My practice runs during dark predawn mornings were often marred by passersby on motorcycles who whistled at me or made a rude comment. Cars would come dangerously close and then whiz away, their drivers delighted at their own playfulness. Solitary men taking a morning walk or making their way to work would stop and stare. I was terrified. Every morning, I would set out wondering if I would be safe that day. I took to walking instead of running—you attract less attention that way, but it didn't help my training at all.

I ran that "Dream Run" anyway. We all completed it, stopping to speak to television crews, hand out Samaritans publicity leaflets with the helpline number, and answer questions from fellow runners and bystanders. The run was a huge success. The effort was a huge boost to my nonexistent athlete ego. I had taken part in a marathon; who would have thought that possible?

Months later in the U.K. as I held the little blue leaflet with the three funny women runners on the logo, I was reminded of the rush of adrenaline, the touch of my feet on tarmac, the pride I felt in completing a race. A women-only group sounded like a good place to start. Plus, they welcomed novices.

The next Tuesday evening I was at the local YMCA along with twenty other beginner runners—each petrified of what we had gotten ourselves into. The beginners were welcomed by Sue Hewett and Jess Wingrove, local women who had been running for many years. The rules were laid out: we would take it slow, stick together, and the runners at the front would "peel back" often to the back, ensuring that everybody stayed together and that there would be no stragglers.

This was not a group for racers. I liked them already.

That evening, in the chilly April breeze, twenty-two women of all shapes and sizes pounded the streets. Focused on the instructions being given, we didn't notice our shortness of breath, the ache in our calves, the rapidly dropping water levels in our bottles. We didn't realize that we had been running for almost forty-five minutes and had covered 2.5 miles. I was dog tired by the time the evening ended. It felt great.

I was back the next Tuesday. And the Tuesday after that. I went on solo runs and on others, accompanied by fellow Sisters. I graduated from being a novice to someone who took pride in being an "older" sister—one who had been around. I wore my blue T-shirt with élan and invested in custom training shoes. I participated in local races, ran London's favorite 5K for women, and was a part of the Running Sisters' Silver Jubilee Race. The medals from those races are my pride and joy.

I cherish the memory of those cold, dark, and very wet Tuesday evenings where, except for the sound of our feet on pavement, nothing stirred. On days like those, we passed by houses, warm and aglow, past schools closed for the night. We ran in rain and in light snow. And when summer came, we breathed in the still cold, but pleasant, sunshine and we were grateful for the light.

In the three years that I ran with the Sisters, not once was I subjected to any kind of harassment or intimidation. There were no whistling, lewd comments, or any attempts by a passerby to touch me. Not once. After my experiences in Mumbai, that felt like heaven. It was so incredibly liberating to choose a route, take a random turn or run in the woods, and know that I was relatively safe. Braving the cold was worth that exhilaration.

Today, I am back in India and I think back on those days with great fondness. With a brand new baby and the monsoons in full swing, I haven't run in a long time. Every time I log on to Facebook, though, my fellow Sisters are there, a reminder of the freedom that I left behind in England, as tangible as the sweat on my brow.

It hasn't happened yet, but I will run again. My running shoes are laced up and waiting where I can see them. They are a constant reminder of how far and how fast I could run and what that jog could do for my body and my self-esteem. I will run again. Maybe tomorrow. Maybe next Tuesday. Tonight, when the baby wakes every few hours, I'll look at those shoes with half-closed eyes and say to myself, *maybe tomorrow, maybe next week, but I will run again.*

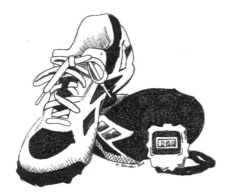

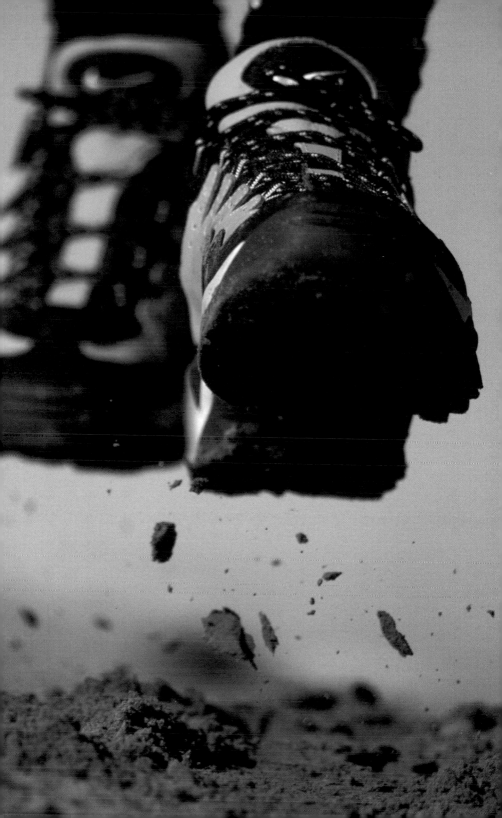

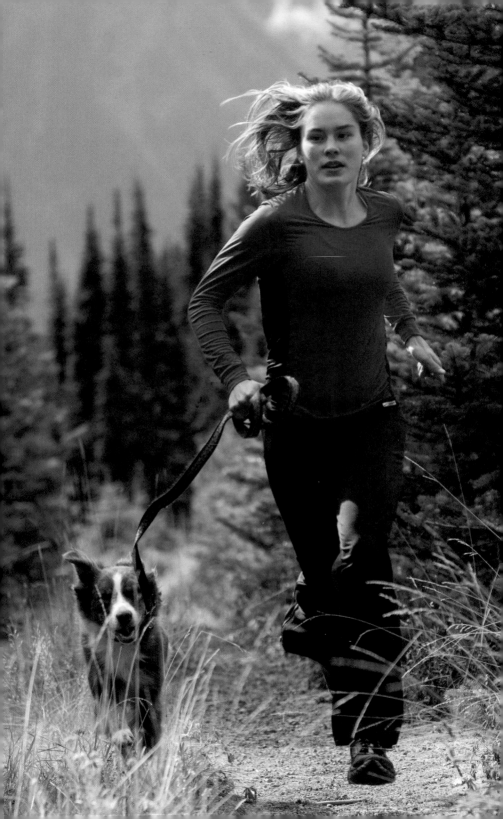

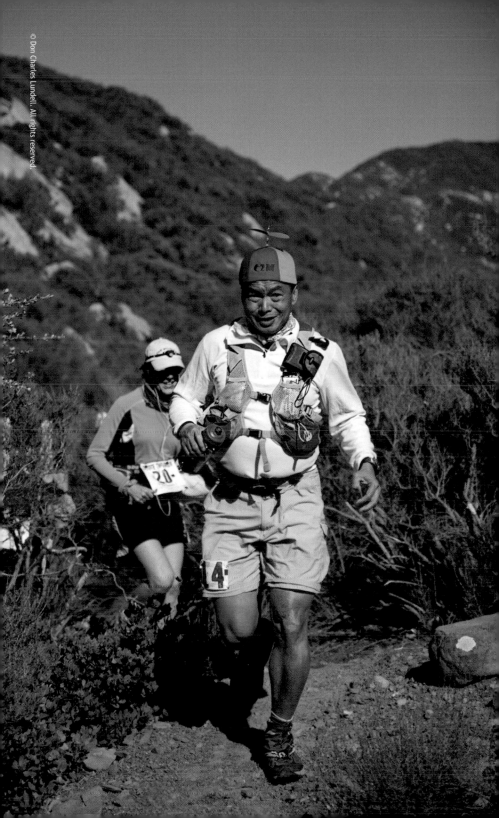

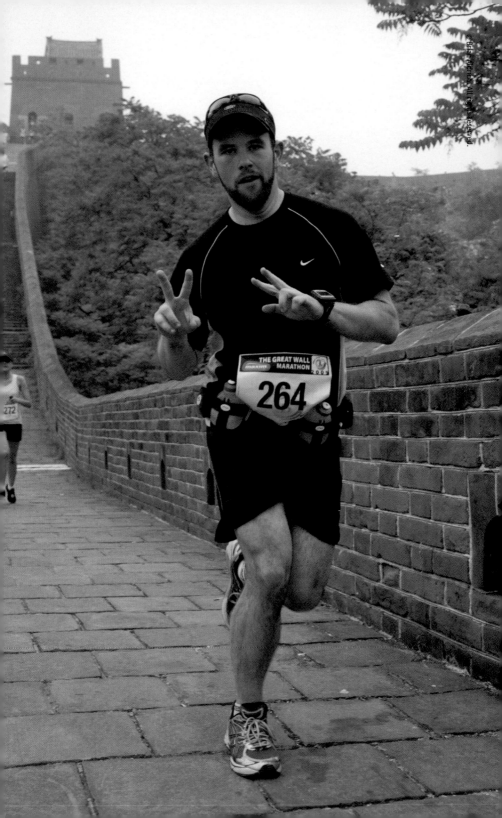

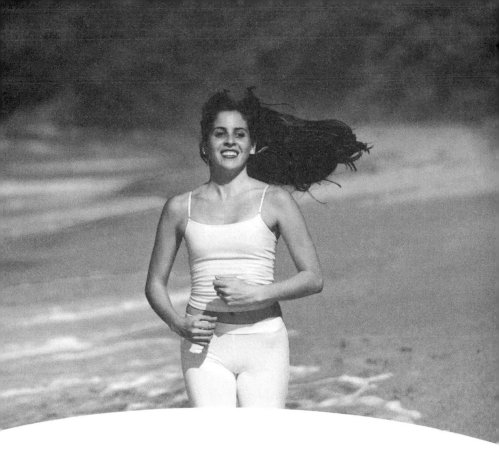

Off the
Beaten Path

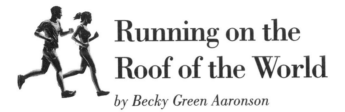

Running on the
Roof of the World

by Becky Green Aaronson

I don't know whether it's the altitude or the view, but the adrenaline surging through me tells me this is one run I will never forget. As I traverse the rocky terrain, I find it impossible to tear my eyes away from the sheer north face of Mount Everest looming in front of me.

I've finally made it to the Roof of the World, and as I run in the shadow of the world's highest mountain, my pounding heart and burning lungs assure me of the 17,000-foot elevation. The thin air and desolate landscape are intoxicating.

Nestled high in the Himalayas, Tibet cast a spell on me like no other place in the world. Not only did it capture my imagination with its ancient Buddhist rituals and colorful Himalayan culture, it also seemed the perfect place for this marathon runner to give herself a new challenge. Knowing that I'd probably never scale Mount Everest, running at Mount Everest Base Camp and other points in between seemed the next best thing.

My adventure began when I met my best friend and former college roommate, Janet, in the Los Angeles airport. Leaving our husbands and responsibilities behind for several weeks, we decided to treat our adventurous souls to what we hoped would be one of many "Girlfriends' Trips of a Lifetime." After a grueling flight over the Pacific, we landed in Hong Kong, then flew to Chengdu, China, the next afternoon before continuing on to Lhasa, Tibet, the following day.

Inside the airport, our guide and driver greet us and place *kathaks* (ceremonial white scarves) around our necks, then whisk us to Lhasa in a Land Cruiser. We'll come to know this four-wheel drive intimately over the next ten days as we travel more than 600 miles on dirt roads from Lhasa to Mount Everest, then on to Kathmandu, Nepal.

After being dropped off at our hotel, we spend the next few days exploring the city. Although I live and run at 8,000 feet, I don't attempt to run here for several days so I can acclimate and avoid altitude sickness in the world's highest capital.

It isn't until the third day, with early morning light brushing the Potala Palace (the Dalai Lama's former home), that I finally set out on my first run. Humbling is the only way to describe it. After running a mile around Potala Square, I'm gasping for air. Each leg feels like it has a twenty-pound bag of cement attached. *Am I getting high-altitude dementia and not remembering that I've done major speed work?* Nope. It's my first attempt at running on the Roof of the World, and it's kicking me square in the pants.

Though my ego is bruised and my body is tired, I feel remarkably energized by the day's activities unfolding around me. A Tibetan couple donned in matching teal and fuchsia workout gear cruises by, waving enthusiastically. They're the only runners I see on this entire trip. While cooling down and stretching my rigor mortis legs, an elderly onlooker praises me in broken English, "You very healthy," which makes my cheeks tickle as I try not to laugh out loud. Based on my performance moments ago, I think, *something MUST be lost in translation.*

After several days of exploring Lhasa's many extraordinary temples, palaces, and monasteries, we set out on our drive across Tibet with Mr. Pei Zhan, our Chinese driver, and Mr. Nobu Tsering, our Tibetan guide-interpreter. Our first day consists of a 150-mile trip from Lhasa to Gyantse. The route takes us over the summit of Kamba-la Pass at nearly 16,000 feet, then drops us down along the shores of holy Yamdrok Lake before delivering us to Gyantse.

The drive to the top of the pass is hair-raising as Mr. Zhan confidently traverses the windy one-lane gravel road with drop-offs of over 1,000 feet and no guardrails to protect us. It doesn't matter if we approach a hairpin curve or a top-heavy cargo truck filled with people and goods; he powers on. My right hand soon becomes permanently attached to the overhead handle by a white-knuckle "death grip." And with no seatbelt, my legs and abdominal muscles take on the job of bracing me as we whip around switchback after switchback.

Janet's eyes are as big as saucers, which is all it takes to send me into a fit of laughter—which in turn, of course, is all it takes to send her into one, too. When she elbows me and whispers, "Maybe we should get out our prayer wheels and start spinning them for good luck," our hysteria crescendos and causes Mr. Zhan's eyes to flash at us in the rearview mirror. Trying not to insult our driver, we take deep breaths and make a pact not to look at each other. Instead we focus out the window.

The view at the top of Kamba-la Pass more than makes up for the drive. Prayer flags flutter in the wind and frame Yamdrok Lake, sprawling out for miles below. The vastness of this high desert landscape reminds us of our insignificance.

When I tell our guide Nobu that I want to get out and run, he and Mr. Zhan look at me like I am mentally ill. Joking that I'm a crazy American, I convince them to stop the car and meet me at the bottom of the road several miles down.

From the first step I take, I know this run is different than any I've ever experienced. The steep descent and roaring tailwind carry me into the clouds as the turquoise waters of Yamdrok Lake transport me to a "running place" I've never been. Step after glorious step and filled with adrenaline, I breathe in joy so deep that my body feels weightless, as if I've sprouted wings. A lightbulb suddenly goes off in my head: *I am, at this very moment, living my favorite Tibetan proverb, "Pain Exists to Measure Pleasure."* Yesterday's humbling schlog in Lhasa was meant to make me fully appreciate the run I'm experiencing right now. I've never felt so alive.

Near the bottom, I spot the waiting Land Cruiser and try to think up any excuse to keep running. Knowing that Nobu and Mr. Zhan have already been patient with me, I reluctantly settle back into my seat, and the thrill of Kamba-la Pass settles deep into my soul.

After arriving in Gyantse in the late afternoon and overnighting, we set out for Shigatse the next day, just two hours away. Although few things Tibetan are left in Shigatse since China erected modern prosaic buildings and wide boulevards, one remaining jewel is Tashilhunpo Monastery, one of the few monasteries to survive the Cultural Revolution.

Instead of running in Shigatse, Janet and I hike the pilgrim trail circling Tashilhunpo. It's a steep path lined with prayer flags and prayer wheels, mani stones, and boulders painted with brightly-colored buddhas. We watch in amazement as elderly pilgrims breeze by us effortlessly, spinning their prayer wheels and greeting us with a warm, *Tashi delek* (hello).

The next day, we make our way toward Mount Everest. Although we're accustomed to being bounced around by now, the drive to Base Camp takes that to new heights. On several occasions our heads brush the roof of the car and our stomachs follow right behind.

As we round the last corner and arrive at Rongbuk Monastery where we'll bunk for the night, a chill shoots through me. The sheer north face of Mount Everest is towering in the distance. As we stand at Base Camp among tents and prayer flags, the mountain's power makes my skin tingle. I'm in awe of the adventurers who'd dare take on this unforgiving 29,000-foot beast.

The twitter in my stomach tells me it's finally my turn to test my mettle at Everest. Even though my version pales in comparison —a five-mile run back to the monastery—it still takes some *major* convincing before Nobu and Mr. Zhan disappear in the Land Cruiser.

As I make my way back from Base Camp, the lack of oxygen immediately makes breathing a challenge and sends my heart rate soaring, but the adrenaline surging through my veins leaves me in a rhythm akin to a celebration. Every step is a gift and every breath a shout out to the country that has wrapped itself so warmly around me. I hear Tibetans' sweet sing-songy voices float through my head as my legs propel me forward. And I visualize their long black hair twisted with colorful yarn, and their naturally happy eyes laughing as we try yak butter tea for the first time. My pounding heart reminds me of the sacred drums we've heard in Tibet's holy temples, and my heavy breathing imitates the sonorous tones of chanting monks. There isn't a moment of this run that I don't appreciate all that Tibet has given me—most of all, the opportunity to experience something extraordinary.

Back at the monastery guesthouse, we're supplied with an endless cup of jasmine tea. My run has caught up with me and I can barely keep my eyes open as I eat my meal by the fire and listen to the sound of yak bells clanking outside. A dull altitude-headache has also set in, so I head off to bed to let my body recover.

The next morning we spring out of bed before dawn and hike back to Base Camp to take pictures of Everest at first light. Even though we're wearing six layers, the blasting wind cuts right through us and leaves us numb. It isn't kind to my camera either. After just one frame my batteries freeze and end my picture taking.

It's a blessing though. Instead of focusing my energy on capturing the changing light on the mountain, I spend it doing something that will forever be etched in my memory. With the jet-stream trail blasting off Everest's north face and the sun's rays splashing down on me, I run along the desolate landscape of Base Camp one last time. The energy radiating from Everest is electric. While jumping over small ice fields and frolicking in Tibet's intoxicating air, the Sanskrit word *namaste* keeps playing over and over in my head. . . . *The spirit in me meets the same spirit in you.*

This is what my running adventure on the Roof of the World has been all about. I may not have scaled Mount Everest, but my spirit has been stirred, and I have been reminded that running will always take me beyond the ordinary.

Namaste, Tibet.

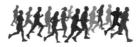

What More Do You Need?

by Mary Monaghan

I rolled over in bed and checked the alarm clock: 5:30 AM. Already light outside and not too hot, a perfect time to run. I pushed the mosquito net aside and reached for my running gear that I'd laid out on a chair the night before. I went to the window, pulled back the curtain, and looked out. What a perfect scene: clear blue skies, palm trees swaying in the wind, and the vivid blue of the Indian Ocean in the distance. I smiled to myself. What a privilege to be here on the coast of Madagascar and to be paid for being here; how lucky I am, I thought.

I had arrived in Madagascar a few weeks earlier to work on a project. It all seemed so exotic and exciting to work on an island known for its natural beauty. I had been warned that life there could be challenging—it was a country of extreme poverty, poor sanitation, and a high risk of malaria. I had to be careful what I ate and drank, but it was a small price to pay for the opportunity to live and work in one of the most beautiful and unspoiled parts of the world.

I quickly put on my running gear and stepped out onto the veranda to check the temperature. Even though it was still early it was already in the 80s: hot, bright, and humid. I gulped down some bottled water and headed down the hill toward the sea. The dusty streets were full of people walking, many carrying buckets on their head as they went to collect water, others walking to the local market with meat or vegetables in wheelbarrows. It was noisy and chaotic. There were very few cars attempting to negotiate the potholed streets; any cars that were there were ancient, rusted, dented, and overcrowded with passengers, barely able to climb any hills they encountered.

I picked my way through the crowds, greeting people as I ran past. They were all very friendly with wide, welcoming smiles for this stranger in their town. I certainly didn't blend in well with them as I was freckled with red hair and I towered above them. Most of them were barefoot in clothes that had been washed and rewashed so many times their vibrant colors were long gone.

I continued my run up the hill toward the lookout point above the sea. After struggling to run in the heat, my face red from exertion, I finally arrived at my destination. It was so beautiful, lush, and green with the darkest of blue seas below—a perfect day. I breathed in the air, clean and fresh, far from any pollution. I watched the goats grazing on the hillside, the palm trees swaying in the light breeze, and counted my blessings for being there on that day and experiencing the joy of running free in such beautiful surroundings.

As I ran on, I spotted a church on a hill above me. I ran toward it, not wanting to go in because I was not dressed correctly but still wanting to investigate a little. I stood outside the door and listened as the congregation started to sing. They had no hymn books, no organ, and yet they sang with an energy, joy, and fervor that I marveled at. There was an exuberance and passion that came straight from the heart. I stood there, my eyes closed, drinking in that moment, feeling their singing touch my soul.

When the singing stopped I continued on my way, feeling humbled by what I had just experienced. I looked down to the sea at the fishermen paddling out in their dugout canoes to check their nets. That's when I bumped into Niry, the young driver from work who was also out for a run. He greeted me warmly.

"Bonjour Mary, isn't it a lovely day?"

"Yes it is. I'm having the most wonderful run. I've been past the church and listened to the singing; it was so beautiful." But even as I said the words, I couldn't help feeling troubled by the sheer poverty I was seeing—the shacks, the rags, the difficulty of daily life.

I asked him, "Do people here not want to get away to the city to earn more money?"

He seemed genuinely surprised by my question. "What more could they need?" he asked. "They fish and use the fish they need for food, then sell the rest and use that money for rice, clothes, and anything else they want. What more could they need?"

I looked down at my expensive running shoes and at Niry's simple ones. He was right, what more could they need? It wasn't necessarily important to have so much. Life here was simple, straightforward, unhurried, nonmaterialistic. It was tough, but that didn't make it bad. I realized I had no right to impose my first-world standards on them. I said good-bye to Niry and set off back to the hotel, stopping by the church to listen again to the joyful singing as it filled the early morning. I had learned a valuable lesson that morning, one that would stay with me for the rest of my life: *What more do you need?*

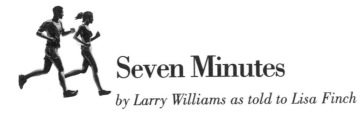

Seven Minutes

by Larry Williams as told to Lisa Finch

It's 5:30 AM, and I lace up and hit the road. I love an early start, when it's still dark out and it's just me and my footfalls on the empty streets. It all belongs to me. Nothing in my way. All worries, all stress, everything gets farther and farther behind me as I move forward.

It wasn't always this way. When I first started, I could barely make it around the block. I have a family history of heart attacks. My older brother Brian passed away at a young age, and I knew that the stress of my job, family life, and just life in general could put me at risk, too. I wanted and needed to get in shape. For me, running is a metaphor for life. If I can reach my goals in running, I can be a better husband, a better father, better at work. Better personally. So I considered training and then doing a marathon. *If I can do that*, I thought, *I can do anything*.

Now here I am, five years later. I've got fifteen races under my belt, ranging from 5K to 50K. Eight of those were 42K. My next full marathon will be my tenth. I could finish with that, knowing that I've met my goal of running ten marathons. But then there's the Boston Marathon.

Seven minutes. That's all that stands between me and the

qualifying time for the Boston Marathon. It isn't the prestige of that particular marathon, although I do admit that has crossed my mind. It's meeting the challenge. My best time to date has been 42K in 3:27. If I can get that down to 3:20, I can do Boston.

When I did my first full marathon, I was amazed at the families carrying signs, even people who weren't related to me, or who didn't know me, cheering, waving, high-fiving, calling my name. At the halfway mark, 20K, I saw my whole family waiting at the sidelines. My wife, Kathleen, our two kids, Nicole and Tyler, some of my in-laws—my family—all waiting for me. And it's the same for me, every race. When all's said and done, no matter who makes it to one of my races, I always know I will see Kathleen, Nicole, and Tyler, if not at the finish, then somewhere along the course, moving me forward. That's how I make it to the finish line.

As a new runner, I dreamed of doing the Around the Bay run in Hamilton, Ontario, a 30K run. It wasn't my first race; in fact it was my ninth. I placed 1,100 out of 3,000; my time was 2:45. But more than the time or my placement, I remember thinking at the end, *I just did Around the Bay!*

You get a lot of time to think when you run. During Around the Bay, we rounded near the cemetery where my older brother Brian was buried. I couldn't help but feel him urge me on to the finish line.

In the Chicago Marathon in 2005, I couldn't concentrate. It was so inspiring to see the buildings, the celebrities, the helicopters. It was almost too much to take in. It took six minutes just to cross the starting line—that's how many people raced with me. There were 41,000 people in that race. And at the end, I was in the top 11,000. I did it.

When I did the ultramarathon in Niagara-on-the-Lake, Ontario in June 2007, I honestly thought at the end I'd pass out. It was a 50K run, and at the 40K mark, my body wanted to quit. I also felt mentally burned out, but I kept going anyway. I saw people passing out, giving up, hitting a wall they just couldn't beat, and I kept on going. I've seen people quit as early as the 5K mark because their time wasn't good. I always think, *This could just be a bad point in their run; it could all turn around and they could get their time back if only they keep going.* Thoughts like that keep *me* going.

It's not a pretty sport, that's for sure. Sometimes it's sheer agony, especially seeing others fall by the wayside. I remember one time, doing a 20K, my legs on fire and completely exhausted, I asked myself, *Why am I doing this?* Then I thought how much it had cost me physically to get there, how much time I'd invested, and I moved forward. Another time, I had injured my leg at work (my kids said it was "gushing blood," but really, it wasn't that bad). Besides, I knew I could still run, if I put my mind to it. If I let a little injury stop me, what other reasons would I find not to run? You can *always* find a reason not to run. But you have to move past that, just like you do when you hit that point during a race.

At some point during every marathon, I know I'm going to hit a wall. It's just a matter of where I'll hit it. But I also know I'll get my second wind afterward. At that point, all the cheering and hoots and hollers fade into the background. All I see are the smiling faces of my kids and my wife. And that's where I'm headed.

Will I make Boston? Seven minutes stand between me and that race. In one sense, it's a short amount of time. But to qualify for Boston, it's everything. I'm going to go for it. There's only one direction in this sport anyway: forward.

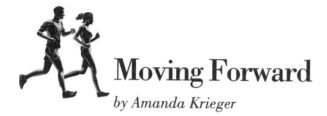

Moving Forward

by Amanda Krieger

I'd gone running here hundreds of times. My feet were on the same pavement, passing the same buildings, navigating the same course. This time, though, something was starkly different.

It wasn't the air hanging heavy in my lungs, and it wasn't the unseasonably cold weather—flurries in mid-April. The difference was in my heart.

Physically, everything was normal. For once, moving blood and oxygen through my body was the least of my heart's worries. As a runner I can ignore soreness, snowstorms, injuries, and cramps, but the pain of running at Virginia Tech after the tragic shootings on April 16, 2007 was something I could not simply grit my teeth and run through.

Virginia Tech is a safe place; no one can convince me otherwise. Not my countless friends who lectured me on the dangers of running alone at night on a college campus, and not Cho Seung-Hui, who killed thirty-two students and teachers before turning the gun on himself.

I had graduated from Virginia Tech almost exactly three years before the school became nationally known as the site of the worst shooting in United States history. Virginia Tech is on a 26,000-acre campus surrounded by breathtaking trails and rolling pastures. Despite the call of the trail, my favorite run was always right on campus, usually at night. Long after the sun set behind the Blue Ridge Mountains, I darted between buildings, dodged students, and reveled in the moonlit academic landscape.

Somewhere between football games, homework, and sleep deprivation, running almost immediately found its place in my life at Virginia Tech. I still remember my first run as a freshman. Just hours after my mom and dad moved me into my freshman dorm, West Ambler Johnston Hall (the dorm where Emily Hilscher and Ryan Clark were killed), a few friends from high school and I jogged around campus, exploring our new and foreign home. A few nights later I embarked on the campus on my own and discovered a beautiful sanctuary that I somehow missed while walking to classes.

In college I grew from a mediocre high school–miler who was secretly intimidated by the distance of a 5K into a confident half-marathoner and triathlete. The hours I spent on campus in my running shoes were the only times I knew for sure what I wanted to do with my life: I wanted to be a runner.

Now, sitting in my office at a newspaper three hours from Blacksburg, Virginia, the initial news of the shootings hit me like a blow to the knees. I frantically called my brother, a freshman at Tech, and choked on tears as I watched the death toll climb. Just hours later my editor sent me to Blacksburg to cover the story.

Being back on campus amid the mourning students and faculty, the media and the yellow tape, caused stress deeper than any exam ever had. I spent the afternoon focusing on work rather than the reality of what was happening around me. I conducted interviews, took photos, and went to press conferences.

Eventually, though, the sun set on April 16, and once my first round of stories were sent, the reality of the tragedy at my beloved college began to sink in. Before a lump could form in my throat I pulled my hair into a ponytail, slipped on my running shoes, and started running.

That night, forward motion was laborious. In the stillness of campus, where I remembered feeling fast and strong, my legs felt heavy and my muscles burdened. Instead of listening to my reluctant body, I fixed my gaze ahead, determined to take each step. As a large grassy field in the center of campus called the Drillfield came into view, my feet instinctively stopped. The field where students usually play frisbee and pick-up football had been transformed into a vigil site, glowing with the mournful warmth of candles. Suddenly, I couldn't ignore it anymore. The rush of emotion overwhelmed me and I bent over with my hands on my knees. Then, as my breaths turned into sobs, I started running again. Tears streamed down my face as I circled the Drillfield. I was angry to the core and overwhelmed with sadness. I cried for the victims, for the survivors, for the campus, for myself, and I ran because I didn't know what else to do. Soon my weary muscles felt powerful, my breaths were strong, and my steps were sure. As I ran, the strength of my alma mater fueled each step.

I rounded the Drillfield and paused at Norris Hall, where most of the shootings took place. The building was encircled by police tape and patrol cars. My feet slowed but they did not stop. I didn't stop because I couldn't. Virginia Tech taught me about progress and the importance of moving forward. For years the energy I felt on the campus of Virginia Tech and the spirit of the Hokies had fueled my runs. Virginia Tech never let me stop and now, more than ever, stopping was not an option.

When I was a student there, running at Virginia Tech got me through exams, heartbreak, and all of the trials that come with becoming an adult. My runs taught me what the classroom couldn't: that no pain lasts as long as you think it will, that you can go about twice as far as you thought you could. On this day of sadness and destruction, running on the campus taught me that even when everything is going wrong, it *is* possible to be strong.

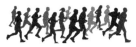

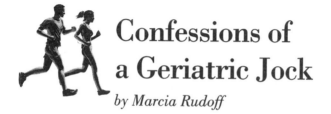

Confessions of
a Geriatric Jock

by Marcia Rudoff

W hat am I doing here? Lazy me, in my sixtieth year, sweating my way through a 5K race, huffing, puffing, and calling myself crazy? What am I doing stumbling up this never-ending hill?

Leonard got me into this. Me, the wannabe couch potato, dreaming of retirement, the easy chair, and the television remote control. Sleeping late, lounging away the day, that's what was supposed to happen when I turned sixty. But no, I had to meet Leonard.

The friends who introduced us said we had so much in common. They never said anything about running races.

When we started dating, his interests seemed normal enough: dinners out, movies, time spent with friends. He never mentioned the R word. What he did say was we should always do things together; it was so much more fun.

Well, you're wrong Leonard. This is not fun.

"You do the 5K while I run the 10K, and then we'll go out for breakfast," he said.

He knows I'm a sucker for breakfast out, or lunch out, or dinner out, or any meal that I don't have to cook. I liked the idea of the breakfast, but I told him I didn't run. "You can walk it," he assured me. Wrong again, Leonard.

Have you ever tried to walk when hundreds of people, packed in around you as far as the eye can see, make the simultaneous decision to run? Picture an ancient, overweight cow attempting a leisurely stroll in the midst of a stampede. I do not walk. I run for my life.

The speedies pull ahead, spread out, and leave me here in their dust. I can walk now—if I can catch my breath and steady my wobbling knees. I'll pace myself: walk a little, run a little, and I'll be fine. I'll make it. Leonard will be proud of me.

I'm running. I've passed three houses, four, ugh, that's enough. I'm winded. Better walk a little more, then run again. Maybe I should rethink this pacing. Instead of walk a little, run a little, I'll run a little, walk a lot. Yes, this is better. Much better. Okay, it's time to trot again.

Ouch, that's enough running; my legs hurt. My pacing still isn't right. How about if I walk until just before they can see me from the finish line and then I run it in looking oh-so-athletic? Let them think I ran the whole thing. How will they know otherwise? I'll be as out of breath and exhausted as the others. The joke will be on them, my revenge for this torture. It's enough to keep me going.

At last, this hill crests! Ah, downhill is better. So much better. I'm easing up. I'm catching my breath. I can even relax enough to look up now, see what's ahead. Another hill, that's what's ahead. Who designs these runs—masochists? What am I doing here anyway? My feet hurt. My legs hurt. My chest hurts. *I* hurt. I want to go home.

A nice level stretch now. They've run out of hills, poor masochistic dears. They must be heartbroken. I'll just keep moving along this even road and the racecourse will have to end soon. It can't go on forever. Everything has to end, doesn't it?

I don't know. I'm beginning to wonder. Maybe this is hell. Maybe I've already expired and been condemned to run this 5K through all eternity.

Oh Lord, forgive me. I repent for all my sins, and I'll never do anything bad again. Just let me see the finish line and I'll be good forever. Please don't let them leave me to die here on the trail. Please let me see my home and loved ones again. Please let me find an easy chair somewhere at the end of all this. It does have an end, doesn't it?

My eyes are running. My nose is running. Even my heart is running, fast. Everything about me is running fast, except me. I'm not running fast. I'm not even running. I'm barely moving. Everyone is passing me. This is embarrassing. How humiliating to be the last one to limp across the finish line.

What if they don't wait for me? Maybe they'll think everyone is in and just pack up and leave and take their finish line with them, and I'll never know where to stop. I've got to hurry. Everyone is getting so far ahead of me. What if they turn a corner and I lose them? I don't know where to go. What if I go the wrong way? Left alone, I always go the wrong way. I've got to hurry. I've got to keep up or be lost forever.

Wait. Someone is slower than me! I can hear him panting behind me. Boy, he's laboring hard. Harder than me. Yeah, I'm not doing so badly.

He's gaining on me though; the panting is coming closer and

closer and, oh dear, he's going to pass me, I can hear it. I'm going to be last again. I just know it, here he comes.

A *dog*? Just a dog, all alone, no runner? I'm being outrun by a big, floppy, stray *dog*? He doesn't even have a race number. I want to go home.

Walk, walk, walk. Sweat, sweat, sweat. That's okay. Sweat makes me look official. Stroll along; I've got this thing licked now. Oh, water station up ahead. Better run a little and impress them. Thank them for the water through huffing and puffing. Oooh, this water's good. And they're cheering for me. *Me*.

"Good going, you can do it, keep it up, you're doing great."

Yes, I am. Hey, I'm in the race; they're just handing out water and encouragement. I *am* good. Real good. Where's that finish line? I'll show them.

Whoa, let's not risk cardiac arrest here. Slow down. They can't see me anymore. Walk now. Walk fast, walk vigorously, but walk. Well maybe run a little. Good pace. Walk a little, run a little, run a little more.

Hey, look at that, up ahead. It's the finish line. Hallelujah! It's still there. They didn't pack it up. They didn't all go home. I'm still in the race. Thank you, Lord, thank you, thank you, and pardon me, Lord, while I run like the dickens across that finish line.

There's Leonard. He's run the 10K, and he's already in. He doesn't even look bushed, the bum.

"Hi Honey. You did it. You finished the whole 5K. I'm so proud of you."

"Yeah, it was fun." Good grief, am I really saying this? Hey, why not. I feel great. When's the next race?

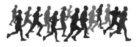

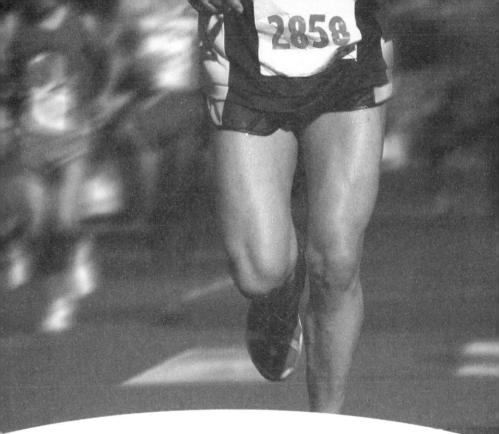

Memorable Races

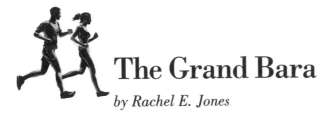

The Grand Bara

by Rachel E. Jones

My grandmother classified me as "the smart one," my younger sister as "the beautiful one," and my older sister as "the athletic one." When my sisters earned their master's degrees and one started medical school (while I could claim a fairly meaningless bachelor of arts), I began to doubt her wisdom in calling me out for my brains. I had already decided she was wrong about my younger sister being the beautiful one—my older sister was equally stunning. And both of them were athletic with race times, trophies, and lean muscles to prove it. But I couldn't shake the feeling that she had been right at least in not labeling me the athletic one. It took a race in the desert of Djibouti for me to prove her wrong.

"You are women," the French soldier said, referring to Lorraine and me.

"Yes, we are," I answered.

"Are you apt?"

"Of course!"

"Are you sure you don't want to ride a bike?"

"We want to run."

"You're civilians."

"But we're apt."

Finally, having agreed that we were apt, the soldier searched through binders and folders and made three phone calls. Although he was the captain in charge of signing people up for the 15K, he didn't know how to sign people up for the 15K. After a fourth phone call, he told me it was too late, sign-up time was over.

"*Si'l vous plait*," I begged, turning on the charm and kissing the captain's cheeks French-style.

And despite the six papers I had to fill out, four *bureaux* I had to visit, and two return visits to the French military base, eventually Lorraine and I were allowed to race. We joined 1,600 French, German, and American soldiers and were among the 100 women to participate.

On race day my husband and I woke up at 3:30 AM to pack the car. We loaded our disgruntled children into the car, still dressed in their pajamas. We picked up another American runner and joined the queue of French soldiers driving into the Djiboutian desert for the annual Grand Bara 15K.

The Grand Bara is so flat and empty, devoid of brush, trees, hills, and valleys, that it is one of the emergency landing sites for a space shuttle. We arrived while it was still dark. A handful of American and French military had camped out overnight, and marching band music blasted from speakers.

When we were called to the starting line, the air was thick with anticipation. A low roar rose from where the morning rays of sun inched along the hills and all eyes turned to the east. Two small lights appeared in the sky and the crowd grew agitated, pointing and shouting.

"Here they come!"

Two fighter jets zoomed over the hills straight at us and the moment they were low, directly overhead, we took off. The adrenaline rush was immediate. Lorraine took about five seconds to lose me in her dust and I pressed on, surrounded by French, German, and American soldiers. The French were polite and silent, the Germans full of laughter and teasing. The Americans were the loudest; running while shouting over their iPods.

The sun rose from behind us and cast a pastel, cloudy sheen over the desert and runners. Body odor steamed from the men, and sweat patches quickly pooled on our shirts as we raced in the heat with no breeze and not a single tree to cast shade over us. The hard, packed clay felt like plush carpet compared to the cement I'd trained on in Djibouti Town.

The desert was silent, other than the pounding of feet on clay and the helicopters overhead, empty and stunning in its desolation. We ran straight, along a row of stones on one side and the wilderness on the other. The highway to Ethiopia ran alongside the rim of the Grand Bara and eighteen-wheelers hurtled to and from Djibouti Town, two hours away. I imagined the drivers staring at the mass of foreigners running in the desert, under a sun that by midday would raise the temperature to one of the highest in the world.

I was fast enough to not be in the last groups but slow enough to miss the orange slices handed out by French soldiers. I did grab a few drinks of water and a sponge of cool water to splash on my head. The water streamed down my face, mingled with sweat, and stung my eyes, but I was grateful for a moment of relief.

My husband and three children were some of the only specta-tors and their cheers spurred me on. Seven-year-old Henry ran with me until he grew tired. The admiration in his eyes as I ran on while he puttered out motivated me to pick up the pace. He didn't know I wasn't supposed to be athletic; no one had ever told him that his mommy wasn't strong or fast.

Two kilometers from the finish I still felt strong. I was tired, but I knew I would finish. I laughed out loud with joy and thank-fulness when it struck me that I had joined my sisters in the ranks of "the athletic ones."

By the time all the racers finished and the French military held an awards ceremony (Lorraine came in second in her age group), the sun beat down on us and the wind had picked up, obscuring the desert and stinging our eyes with dust. We hitched a ride back to our car at the starting line, and I was amazed at how far we had run.

On the way home, we passed a wild ostrich standing motion-less beneath a fifty-foot-high dust devil and surrounded by thorny acacia trees.

I'm with you, Monsieur Ostrich, I thought. *I'm a runner, too.*

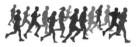

Relentless Forward Motion on the White Line from Hell to Heaven

by Frank McKinney

Badwater Ultramarathon was named by *National Geographic Adventure* magazine as its #1 pick for the world's Top 10 Toughest Races, and the Discovery Channel called it the "world's toughest footrace." I've run Badwater several times—it is a grueling test of endurance and discipline . . . and a spiritual touchstone for me. Running, walking, and dragging myself through this race has been the single best metaphor for living that I've found. Whether you're a runner/athlete or not, you can certainly relate to the ups and downs that so closely mirror life's own triumphs and trials. For me, running and finishing this race multiple times has provided me with some of my most enlightening experiences.

Having Badwater become a part of my being at this stage of my life (I first ran it when I was forty-two years old) has caused me to reflect and then distill the lessons I've learned while chasing the white line from hell to heaven. To run a race like Badwater sounds like an incredible feat to many people—something out there in that blackness beyond the headlights. Often, I hear, "There's no way I could do that, Frank." But they could. I know they could. (The average age of the participants is forty-seven, and the oldest is seventy!) Maybe 135 miles sounds impossible, but could you walk or run *one* mile—and then do it 135 times? Of course! But if you've never done it before, conceiving of the whole thing at once makes your knees knock, at least if you have any sense. Similarly, once you're in that race, it's a death sentence to start thinking about the end when you're only at mile twenty-six (equivalent to a regular marathon) and still have 109 miles in 130-degree heat to the finish. The thing that will keep you going is to focus on *taking the next step,* and on achieving very short milestones, like getting to the next mile marker, or to that cactus just up ahead. You simply have to keep moving forward. In fact, at home I have inscribed directly in front of my treadmill: RELENTLESS FORWARD MOTION. It's one of those truisms that applies not just to physical endurance and excellence, but to business, and to the business of life.

In the Badwater Ultramarathon itself, the goal is no wasted effort; again, it's relentless forward motion. Many people don't finish at all, and I'll tell you why. They start out too fast. They don't pace themselves. They zigzag, crossing the road and wasting steps; they stop to eat and chat and piddle around. At some point, the body gets hyperfatigued and sleep deprived, and since the mental game was lost miles ago, they're out. Since the inception of this epic race in 1977, only about 65 percent of the ninety entrants selected to participate in each race actually finish.

Each footfall across the desert is akin to a rebirthing. The forty-eight hour gestation period leads to a new, raw outlook on life. Your mind shifts, your body cries out, and your soul is cleansed in two days' fire when nothing else matters but your survival, your relentless forward motion, and the people who are supporting you in the race, bringing you water and food and encouragement. Your senses are heightened to a state of euphoria by the majesty of Death Valley.

In 2005, I was invited to my first Badwater. I was the very essence of a rookie; certainly, my resume was the lightest of the ninety-racer field. After a year of intense preparation, self-denial, and self-sacrifice, I endured hellish conditions to finish on July 13, 2005, in 48:49:20. I was never more content and happy in my life, and for a time, I experienced crystalline pure jubilation. I accomplished my goal of finishing the race and told those close to me that I would never return. Lesson: **Never say never to anything in life.** After a few weeks passed, I felt there was something missing from my 2005 experience. Those who finish Badwater in under forty-eight hours are awarded the coveted Badwater belt buckle, the holy grail of ultrarunning circles—and I'd missed earning mine by a mere forty-nine minutes and twenty seconds. If only I had run another 260 feet each hour, I could have had that prize. It didn't matter at the time, and I wish it hadn't mattered after the passage of some time, but it did.

There was only one way to approach my next attempt the following year: intense visualization, meditation, and prayer. My crew and I arrived at the start line on July 24, 2006. With the temperature already exceeding 105 degrees, the gun went off at eight in the morning and I set off in my pursuit of "Sub-48." That was our mantra. We even had team shirts made up that depicted a submarine under water with the number forty-eight on it. I was determined to earn that belt buckle this time.

It didn't begin well. I arrived at the forty-two-mile checkpoint over an hour behind my time from the prior year.

Meanwhile, the race was literally heating up. The mercury soared to 131 degrees. The pavement exceeded 200. One crew-member handed me a peanut-butter-and-jelly sandwich that I carried for a few hundred yards, and by the time I brought it to my mouth, the bread was toasted! By mile fifty I was experiencing severe gastrointestinal problems, and by mile fifty-five I had horrible blisters (I still had eighty miles to go). By mile sixty, while climbing the first 5,000-foot pass, I was running with ice bags on my hips to try to reduce the inflammation. Some twenty hours into the race, I tried to cool down and rest by taking off all my running clothes and lying in the back of the crew van, completely spent. Due to total heat exhaustion, I couldn't focus even a few feet in front of me. My head spun and my body shook. My wife, Nilsa, tells me I attempted to speak but didn't make any sense. At some point, I stumbled out of the van completely naked, body quivering even though it was 108 degrees, crawled on the dirt on all fours, and vomited for half an hour. All fluids were lost, and likely my race was lost, as well.

Drawing from my 2005 ordeal, I knew perhaps with time and faith that this could pass, and I could at least finish. Lesson: **Regardless of the debilitating moments we face in our business, health, personal life, relationships, etc., if we just allow the passage of time and a little faith in God to cure the ailment, often we can emerge ready to conquer.**

At the time, I was unsure if I could continue. I decided to put my shorts and shoes on and start walking very slowly as the sun came up on day two. There was no running at this point, just dragging one foot in front of the other. In this phase of the race, my spirit was nearly broken. While I was dreading another day of blazing heat, something unusual happened. In the middle of the desert, a few dark clouds started to form at mile ninety-five, one just overhead. This cloud stayed with us and, while still hot, protected us from direct sun for hours. It was a gift from heaven.

As we passed the 100-mile mark at 3:30 in the afternoon, we celebrated by having the crew douse me with silly string. With thirty-five miles to go (only a marathon and a half), we were gaining on lost time. We were picking up the pace. I had made it through a very low point.

At mile 105, the sky turned even darker and began to rumble. Lightning was striking within a few hundred yards. Then suddenly a downpour began of a magnitude rarely seen in Death Valley. The raindrops turned to the size of peas and every other one froze into a pellet of hail. Oddly, the temperature dropped to an unbelievable sixty-seven degrees—an incredible relief from the heat.

The hills were unable to absorb the heavy rains. Within thirty minutes, we were engulfed in a full-blown flash flood, where washouts a few feet deep swallowed the road where we continued to run. As we crossed one intense washout I decided to do what probably no other runner in the history of the race has done, to "swim Badwater." I dove into the current as it passed over the road and actually swam for a few minutes. Now, we were having fun. I'd never felt better.

The rains stopped as quickly as they came. As the daylight hours waned on day two, I was rockin' to heavy metal on my MP3 player while I sprinted with a friend—yes, *sprinted*—across the desert, singing and throwing stuff. We still had a full marathon to go, but I don't think I ever had more fun running in my life as I did in the last three to four hours of daylight on July 25, 2006. For the last thirteen miles of the race, I wondered, *Could I make it?* The elevation climbed from 2,500 to 8,500 feet—this after I'd endured 122 miles. *Would we cross the finish line in under forty-eight hours?* All of the excitement of the storm and the sprinter's pace of a few hours before had completely sapped my energy. I was not used to the elevation, and I began to get very dizzy and short of breath. The pressure on my blistered feet was magnified by the steepness of the grade. My feet were now bleeding, but no way was I going to risk stopping and perhaps cramping. At a pace of two miles per hour, I trudged toward the finish line. It was well after midnight, and there were so many stars that there was more white than black in the sky. When we had only a few miles to go, the temperature dropped again, and I was in the midst of a slow death march. Finally, around what seemed to be an unending number of switchbacks came a faint glow that grew brighter as we approached.

Could it be?

It was the finish line.

Our entire crew and my daughter, Laura, and my mom, Katie, joined us for the final sprint to the line. With tears streaming down our faces, we broke the tape as a team. It was the team who got me there, and they were going to finish with me, all eight of us together.

I fell to my knees, overcome with emotion. I looked at my watch, and yes, after nearly two years of training and sacrifice it read 43:02:40! I crushed it by nearly six hours over the year before! The hard work, the desire, the passion, and self-denial resulted in meeting the most significant personal challenge and achievement of my life so far. Lesson: **Life's pursuits are always about the journey, not the destination.**

As I've said before, we all have our own Badwaters, our own goals and aspirations that lay themselves on our hearts. They pierce mere desire and result in passionate and "tunnel-visioned" pursuit. Are you willing to understand and commit totally to whatever your Badwater represents? Relentless forward motion. Creative persistence and perseverance. Never giving up and giving the pursuit enough time to produce the desired results. My life's aspirations may be nothing like yours, yet any and every time you take the incomprehensible and turn it into the possible, the same kinds of dedication and courage are required. Whatever the "incomprehensible" thing is, everyone goes through peaks and valleys, the dry desert and the lush mountains. Everyone has the opportunity either to respond or to turn away. Everyone has the choice of seeking out the familiar and the comfortable and the mundane and the unfulfilling—or to face their fears and go for it.

At the end of any "race," you may say, "Never again!" The pain may be great. You may be exhausted. But then time passes, and you have faith, and the will to run can come back again. You're called to focus on the best and brightest, not to languish in your past, most desperate moments. As you run the next race, keeping your mind on what makes you strong, confident, and moving forward will propel you down the road.

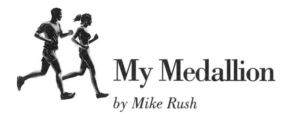

My Medallion

by Mike Rush

"Hey, Bekah, look at this," I said to my oldest daughter, Rebekah, who was a seventh-grader. We were standing in front of the bulletin board that hung outside the laundromat, and I was reading the flyer that announced the Freeze Your Buns Off 5K.

"That looks like fun," she replied.

"Do you want to do it? It's next month, in February, and it'll be cold. Do you think you can make yourself run with me?"

"Yeah, let's do it," she said. "We'll get to be together."

And so it was decided. We would run five kilometers in the freezing cold beginning at 6:30 AM. That's probably why the race was called the Freeze Your Buns Off 5K. The poster promised two things for every runner: a sense of accomplishment and a package of hot dog buns.

I had a mental picture of us on race day: a pair of slender bodies striding rhythmically together, the breeze ruffling the edges of our sleek nylon shorts and jerseys. Our running would be characterized by long, inaudible steps, our hair in graceful waves behind us, our faces trained on the road ahead. The first training run together proved to be anything but idyllic. I finally let go of my vision for us; we would simply jog as much of the three miles as we could and walk the rest.

We were living in the Netherlands at the time. Bekah was playing her first year of youth-league basketball. I loved watching her play, but we really couldn't connect through her basketball experience. I'd never played organized basketball, but more important, her coach was the "other" man in her life. I missed being her only adult male friend.

On the day of the race, I was up early to get us ready and out the door. It was especially cold that morning, just as the flyer had promised. We *were* going to freeze our buns off.

Arriving a few minutes before the start, we joined the crowd of nearly twenty runners forming at the entrance to the military base where the race would be held. We received our instructions from a burly military man.

"You'll run through the gate and down the entrance road. Take the first left; run through the village and up the hill. Take a left at the "T" and follow that road around the back of the base. You'll come down next to the railroad tracks. Just follow them back to the gate here; the finish line will be just inside. When we're all back we'll meet in the fitness center."

The other runners had sleek and slender bodies, just like the ones I'd seen in my vision. Bekah and I, on the other hand, didn't look like serious runners. We wore so many layers we looked like Bibendum, the Michelin Man character, and his daughter. Bekah completed this awkward look with mittens and a ski cap.

I felt a little out of place as the gun sounded. I was the only teacher there; the rest of the runners were military personnel, and they all seemed to know each other. I was also the only person to bring a child. What had seemed like such a great idea six weeks ago was now unfolding as a great opportunity for embarrassment. Bekah and I fell behind the pack just outside of the gate. And just as we reached the halfway point to the first turn, the last of the runners ahead rounded the corner, disappearing from view.

"Dad, I have to walk. I'm sorry."

Her words jabbed at my heart.

"That's okay baby, this isn't about setting a record or anything. Let's just have fun and be together."

"I know, but you'd probably be running if I hadn't come. We're going to be the last ones to finish. It's going to be embarrassing."

"Bekah, that doesn't mean a thing. I love you and I wanted to run with you. That's the most important thing to me."

We jogged some more, made the left turn, and then walked most of the way up the hill. When we reached the flat slope at the top, we jogged again. Our talk turned to school and the excitement of Bekah being my math student the following year. As we slowed to walk again, a young American man approached us on a bike.

"Are you two in the race?"

"Yes," I replied, "is there a problem?"

"No, they just wanted me to check on you. A few people have finished, and you're pretty far back."

I wondered how this made Bekah feel, but she didn't let on that it bothered her. And suddenly I understood the deeper meaning of the two of us being out here, jogging, walking, freezing, but together. I took her hand, and through lips so cold they could hardly move I said, "Bekah, I'm so glad we did this."

"I am, too, Dad," she said, and then the air filled with snowflakes.

We crossed the finish line and made our way to the fitness center. The guy who had given the announcements at the beginning of the race was standing, once again, in front of the crowd.

"We've got medallions for the first and second finishers in each age bracket."

Bekah and I suppressed a giggle. The last runner had finished almost twenty minutes before we did. We probably would have left, but we weren't about to walk away from the hot dog buns we'd frozen our own buns off to earn.

We watched the first five winners receive their medallions. One more, and the only thing between us and home was a bag of buns.

"And the second place medal in the women's C-class goes to Rebekah Rush."

I couldn't believe my ears. There must have been only two runners in Bekah's class. Applause and cheers accompanied her to the front. I watched in awe as the medallion was hung around her neck. When she turned around, I swear her smile lit up the room. I hugged her when she got back to me. She put the medal in front of my face so I could get a better look, and I just shook my head and hugged her again.

While we had been distracted, concluding remarks were said and everyone started for the door, grabbing their hot dog buns on the way out. A few minutes later, we were on our way home.

"Bekah, I'm so proud of you!" I said. "You hung in there and finished."

"But Dad, you don't have a medallion."

Her concern for my feelings touched me so deeply I had to steady my breathing.

"Oh Bekah, don't you understand? *You* are my medallion."

"I love you, Dad."

A View from the Rear of the Miami Half Marathon

by Joseph F. Rottino

I remember well those days when once I was a runner; certainly not an elite or, for that matter, a very good one, but a runner nevertheless. Those were the days of sub-four-hour marathons and twenty-minute 5Ks. Fifteen years, fifteen pounds, and a few nagging injuries certainly make a difference. Or as Hamlet said in his famous "To be or not to be" soliloquy, "Who would bear the whips and scorns of time." The following are illustrative statistics: 1993 Bay Shore (New York) Half Marathon, 1:37:30, versus 2008 Miami Half Marathon, 2:48:28. For the mathematically inclined, that's a loss of about seventy minutes. I no longer run long or fast. I now plod, amble, jig, list, run a few, walk a few, but am happy just to put one foot in front of the other.

However, there are compensations. As a nonrunner, I've become more outward-directed, not overly concerned with pace, splits, and form, although I still wear a stopwatch, which I consult at mile markers and in between. Old habits die hard. I now strike up conversations with those about me and really observe the courses on which I find myself.

So, gentle reader, let me tell you of my triumphs and misfortunes in Miami on January 27, 2008. Actually, my story begins the day before when I drove to Miami Beach to pick up my race packets for a 5K on Saturday and Sunday's half marathon. After exiting my car in the parking lot, I noticed a white pickup truck careening around a corner and seconds later careening into me. The sucker had hit me in the parking lot of the Miami Beach Convention Center. Luckily, I was able to cushion the blow and with my hands repel myself from his left front fender. But he did catch my right knee, leaving a large scrape which eventually scabbed over.

"Are you okay?"

"No, thanks to you. What the hell are you doing?"

"I never saw you."

"That's because you're having a conversation on your cell phone."

"I'm sorry."

"Slow down, or the next person you hit might be a lawyer."

Talk about auspicious beginnings. After my near brush with destiny, I entered the expo where I bought some equipment and T-shirts I didn't need. Then, I ran into Erica Gassen and Anne Anderson, two old running friends from Long Island, who I always meet at the expo, the subsequent 5K on Saturday, and half on Sunday. It's like a given in a geometry proof that our paths will cross on this weekend. And, indeed, our paths did cross again at the end of the 5K in which Erica garnered a second place and I, a fifth-place age-group medal. I had run this race for the past three years because it's a good predictor of the next day's half or full marathon. It began at Watson Island, the one-mile split of the longer races, traversing the MacArthur Causeway to the vicinity of the Nikki Beach Club located at the four-mile marker. As I tried to run the race in my nonrunning style, I predicted that I would not appear on that course the next day. My legs sunk in concrete, my lungs bursting, I felt I couldn't possibly cover the distance on Sunday. I limped across the finish line with an all-time PR (personal record) of 36:23—disgusted with my effort and completely discouraged with my chances of finishing a half marathon anywhere at anytime.

When I got home, I told my wife that I couldn't possibly run the next day.

"But you won a medal in the 5K," she countered.

"Only because everyone in my age group was hospitalized, incapacitated, or dead," I replied.

So I spent the day secure in my decision to bag the half. But that evening I started thinking of my runner friend Howard Kestenbaum. *Here's a guy*, I thought, *who is nearly seventy-seven years old and going to run the full marathon, a month or two after completing another one. What kind of fraud am I not to at least try to do this race, given Howard's determination and pluck?* So, inspired by this stalwart septuagenarian, I set the alarm for 3:00 AM the next morning. I was back in the field.

I left my apartment at 3:45 AM on Sunday and stopped off at the local 7-Eleven for coffee. At about this time, three creatures of the night dragged themselves into the store looking to buy some beer. Too bad it's past the curfew. But I did find myself in a conversation with one of the thirsty trio.

"Say, you look like you're going running."

"That's right. I'm doing a half marathon in Miami."

"No kidding. What's going on."

"It's the Miami Marathon and Half Marathon."

"How come you're up so early?"

"The race begins at 6:00 AM."

"Man, that's early. By the way, how old are you?"

"Seventy."

"No way!"

"Yes, seventy-one next month."

"You're putting me on."

"No, seventy it is."

"Man, that's impressive. You know what. I'm going to stop smoking. Good luck in the race."

"Thanks."

So having opened the possibilities of a healthier lifestyle to my new friend, I proceeded to Miami, where at 6:00 AM I found myself with some five thousand runners waiting for the gun to start the race. Moments later, I smelled the unmistakable aroma of marijuana drifting toward me. I turned to the right and saw a young lady taking a large toke of, can you believe it, a *joint*. As the smoke wafted out onto the morning air, the crowd around her started to chant, "Share, Share, Share." After saving one poor soul from the ravages of nicotine, I have lost another to the chains of cannabis.

The gun finally went off and the night was lit by a starburst of multicolored fireworks: yellows, whites, greens, reds, and pinks brightened the dark sky. It took me some two and a half minutes to reach the start line. As the crowd surged around me, I started to run. At the half-mile mark, I found myself walking up one of the few elevations in the race on the causeway to Miami Beach. To the right was fabulous Port of Miami with its myriad ocean liners. The ships were ablaze as strings of lights outlined those immense floating palaces of pleasure. Foghorns and sirens blasted through the early morning silence, urging the runners to run the best race they could and enjoy the magnificent course.

I covered the causeway in my lurching run-walk style, not knowing if I would be able to complete the race. After hundreds of long-distance training runs and races ranging from half marathons to 100 kilometers, I was doing this on memory. My long runs in the past four months had been six, maybe seven miles. But as I wandered on, I was fascinated by the diverse characters that comprised the rear of the pack. This was no homogenized group of trim, lean endomorphs found among the leaders of the race. Runners of all shapes, sizes, colors, and ethnicities ran alongside me. Large women, frail men, the lame, the halting, and even the blind somehow managed to find the wherewithal to compete in this physical contest. It was indeed a testament to their courage and determination. At mile three, I came across a heavyset woman on a hand-crank bike, sweating and straining to reach the top of a rather long upgrade on the causeway. After cresting the hill, she went into freefall on the way down, barely missing runners who scrambled out of the way as she streaked toward the Miami Beach peninsula. Later on at mile ten, I met a young woman who was running, not walking, with a cane supporting her. I called her "my hero." She smiled and promised to meet me at the finish line. Her grin widened when I told her she'd have to wait for me, even as I pulled ahead. Although we would never hook up, I was warmed by our chance encounter.

At mile four, the course reached the lower tip of Miami Beach where it makes a U-turn at Joe's Stone Crab, a famous landmark restaurant, and past the now silent, but usually swinging Nikki Beach Club. It was at this point that Erica Gassen waved at me from the crowd of bystanders and took my picture. I was delighted to see her again. She told me that I was a few minutes behind fellow Long Island runner Carl Grossbard, whom I later met at the finish line to share running stories and postrace refreshments. At this point in the race I was feeling strong, having settled into a rhythm of sorts after the ragged breathing and heavy-leg syndrome that had characterized my earlier efforts.

I marveled at a runner who was running and simultaneously juggling three balls as I proceeded up Ocean Drive. The sun had now risen and I glimpsed it shining off the calm ocean. After grabbing a cup of water at mile five, I started a conversation with Leroi, a large gray-bearded African American gentleman who told me that he was running his first half marathon because his wife had persuaded him that running would keep him healthy. Unfortunately, his wife, with whom he was supposed to run today's event, was home sick in bed with a fever. We immediately found common ground—jazz. We swapped stories and I told him of musicians I'd seen perform and spoken to in nightclubs and concert halls from Philadelphia to Boston; musicians including Louis Armstrong, Red Allen, and Count Basie. I talked about legendary cafes I'd frequented in New York during the fifties and into the seventies: Nick's, Eddie Condon's, and Birdland, to name a few, from the Village, Uptown, and into Harlem. He was familiar with the names and places I mentioned and told me of his similar experiences. We agreed that those days, now long gone, were wonderful, and we are saddened by their passing.

Leroi's pace slowed and I left him at mile nine having spent a delightful four-mile interval with a kindred spirit, where the rigors of the race were secondary to the stimulating shared conversation. Just as I left Miami Beach at mile eight, the field was encouraged by the cheerleading squad and drum brigade from Miami Beach Senior High School. It was a welcome pick-me-up as the beat of the drums and the cheers put a spring in my step and brought a smile to my face. I began to cross the Venetian Causeway heading west back to Miami. This is really a series of six drop-dead beautiful islands connected by a set of low bridges. The foliage lining the roadway is lush and tropical with the hint of magnificent homes peeking out from behind the flora.

As I reentered Miami, I passed a spectator zone where a crowd welcomed the racers back to the mainland with cheers, noise-makers, and musical instruments. I was especially taken by a group of scantily clad, extremely sinuous young women who were painted sky blue from stem to stern. They were screaming and yelling, raising the temperatures, heartbeats, and spirits of all who passed by. Somewhere on the causeway, I ran into Charles Vermailon, an old running buddy. We compared our list of aches, pains, and injuries. Charles was nursing a knee that gave out on him earlier in the race when he stepped into a depression on Ocean Drive. (The next time I ran with him, he was wearing a knee brace.) We commiserated with one another; I complained about a chronic pain in my right heel that I had been living with for six months. We settled into a pattern: we ran together, then I stopped to walk, resumed running, caught up and passed Charlie, who then caught and passed me when I stopped to walk.

At mile ten, the course had entered a grittier part of town, sort of an industrial area. Ahead there was a dynamic salsa band turning the race into a Latin dance as I high-stepped by. Turning the corner was another water stop where I spied an absolutely heavenly vision. She was mocha colored with long, dark hair falling to her shoulders; curvaceous, capturing the moment with a startling, gleaming white-toothed smile. I was totally enthralled as I drank the water from the cup she handed me. I told her I wanted to take her home with me instead of the finisher's medal. She laughed, patted me on the shoulder, and sent me on my way with a wistful smile on my face. I figured she had probably received at least two thousand similar proposals already.

At mile twelve, the race turned right at the American Airlines Arena, home of the Miami Heat, and ambled down Biscayne Boulevard, where at mile 12.5 the course split, with the full marathoners heading south into Coral Gables and the rest of us turning left and then negotiating a series of turns to the finish line at Bayfront Park. At this point in the race, there were only a few hardy souls who were running the entire marathon. I shuddered at the thought of having to run some thirteen-plus more miles. I muttered a "Thank God" to myself that I was nearing a finish line, rather than running away from one. And then, there it was. Having just passed through an S-turn, I burst onto the straightaway. There were bleachers on the left, filled with cheering spectators and a finish line some two hundred meters ahead. I went into my sprint mode and passed a few stragglers as I crossed the line. I breathed deeply, steadying myself as my legs started to quiver, and smiled as a finish-line volunteer of unparalleled warmth and charm put a large "gold and diamond-encrusted" spinning medal over my head and onto my chest. I glanced at my watch. I had covered the course in 2:48:28, upward of a 12:50 pace. The time was super slow, but I didn't care. If I had not conquered, I had, at least, endured.

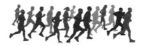

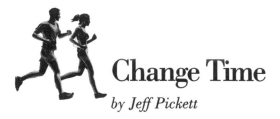

Change Time

by Jeff Pickett

Running is a sport anyone can enjoy. You can start at any age, you can come from any country, and your weight or height don't matter at all. Just getting out and doing it are the only action steps needed. At least, that's what most of us think.

Then there are the insanely crazy people who definitely fall into the "What Were You Thinking?" category. Take, for example, the guy I met at the Chicago Marathon about ten years ago.

It was my first marathon and I was both scared and nervous. The race started, and the crowd merged forward to cross the starting line, which also helped quiet the butterflies in my stomach. Well, some of them anyway. My eyes were taking in all the sights and sounds of the marathon, enjoying the beautiful cityscape of Chicago as it unfolded in a new way, special even for someone who used to live there. I saw many things that day—and soon I would see too much.

At about the six-mile marker, I heard it before I saw it. The sound was unmistakable: the jingle of keys and coins. From the sound of them, there were enough to fill a piggy bank a few times over—or at least start a few hundred cars. I quickened my pace slightly, determined to discover the source of this metallic symphony. If I had only been prepared for the sight that accompanied the sounds. . . .

After peeking at my watch to check my pace, I lifted my eyes and saw a man in his midthirties. His sweatband was askew and his socks were pulled up to about midcalf. I wish now that was all I had seen, but unfortunately I saw much more. The metallic sounds I'd been hearing were definitely coming from this unfortunate soul.

There was no mistake—this guy was a first-timer, like me. However, he was a little more prepared than I was. Much more prepared. Okay, I have to say it: he was overprepared.

Wearing his new RaceReady shorts (you know, the kind that have built-in pockets in back), this man had stashed his entire life savings and every key he could find. You could also see the glint of packaging familiar to marathon runners everywhere; there must have been ten packs of GU protruding from those back pockets. And yet, it got better.

As the coins and keys clinked against each other, the impossible burden of all this weight was doing two things. First, it was undoing some of the seaming on his pockets, which made the GU that much more visible. But in addition, the weight of the keys, coins, GU, and Davy Jones' locker in this man's shorts was also revealing . . . his crack. Now, when you talk about seeing someone's crack, you usually mean exactly that; crack—as in a smidgen or small percentage. But I'll bet at least 50 percent of this man's crack and a sizeable portion of his buttocks were in plain view.

I respected this man as a runner and so I fought the urge to laugh. The guy next to me, however, came from a different school of thought and compassion. Even while running six miles at a nine-minute-per-mile pace, the young guy next to me guffawed like he was at a comedy show. You know how laughter is—one guy starts, others join in, and I have to admit, it made me laugh, too. In fact, I was laughing so hard I had to pass the guy before it blew my focus even more. I didn't plan to add a DNF (Did Not Finish) next to my first marathon attempt.

After what seemed like hours, I finally did pass the gentleman with the protruding crack. I looked over and subtly waved, wondering how on *earth* he could be so oblivious to his "condition." *Doesn't the cool morning air on his rear distinguish itself from the warmth of his upper body? Doesn't he hear the laughter around him?* And I wondered, *How much money exactly did he decide to put in his pockets that morning and what is he going to do with all that change? Who is he going to call? Was he going to stop by the laundromat as soon as his run was finished?* These were all questions I will never know the answer to. To this day I lay awake many a night, just wondering.

Once I was ahead of him, I took a few deep breaths. I could still hear the metallic clinking and I couldn't stop smiling. I felt the sudden urge for a GU myself and reached back in my pack for one. As I ripped off the top and squirted it into my mouth, I was smiling so much I forgot to aim and open my mouth. The thick liquid landed half on my lips and half on my cheeks before dribbling down the front of my shirt. Lovely. Now there was something else for my fellow runners to laugh about.

I completed my first marathon that day. It was a great experience, and I also learned some valuable lessons. The memory of that man and his overloaded shorts will always stick with me. To this day I have never worn RaceReady shorts. I never take coins with me on a run. I lace up my shorts nice and tight. And if I ever hear any laughter during my races, especially from behind me, I'm quick to investigate the exact location of my waistband.

I've been lucky so far. No YouTube videos have surfaced of me and my crack. I plan to keep it that way.

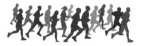

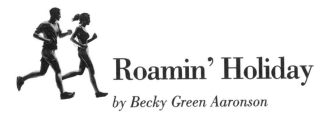

Roamin' Holiday

by Becky Green Aaronson

You know what they say . . . "When in Rome . . ." And as I mingle with other runners at the start of the marathon and ogle at the ancient architecture of the Coliseum, I plan to do just that. Romans and visitors alike join in the countdown, and then take off to the spirited command, *andiamo!*

So begins my *Roman Holiday*—or at least my modern adaptation of this romantic 1950s film classic. While Gregory Peck and Audrey Hepburn motored around the city on a scooter, my version will propel me through the streets on foot as I soak up all things Roman.

The racecourse is a treasure trove for history buffs, and it doesn't take long before my head is spinning. First we run past the Forum, the ancient center of the city. Then we run past the Tomb of the Unknown Soldier and the grandiose marble compound often referred to as the "Wedding Cake," due to its cake-like shape. It's really a nineteenth-century monument to Victor Emmanuel II, king of Italy, but being a newlywed, I find its name amusingly appropriate, and of course think it's plopped on the route just for me. You see, not only have I come to Rome to run the marathon but my husband and I have come to the Eternal

City to celebrate our honeymoon. After I finish the race, he plans to swoop me up like Gregory Peck to go create Part II of our *Roman Holiday*—the romantic part.

After snaking our way along the Tiber River, then passing one historic building after another, I realize that while the landmarks are stunning, it's the *feel* of this marathon that makes it unforgettable. I decide to stop cataloging the monuments in my head and, instead, drink in the flavor and charm of the race.

It doesn't take long before I'm *literally* drinking in a uniquely Roman aid-station staple—*acqua con gas* (sparkling water)— which I choke on, of course, recovering only about a quarter-mile later. Parisians are known for their good humor, serving wine and cheese at some of their aid stations, but Romans obviously have a more slapstick approach. This gag *has* to be designed to see how many *turistas* they can punk. And boy, did they get me good.

As we cross over Ponte Cavour and head toward the Vatican, we cruise past a service that is underway. It makes me feel, how shall I say it—not very pious. This is the first "Sunday Service" marathon I've ever experienced, and I hope the Big Guy is okay with it. Who knows, maybe the pope is sending a cheer our way, or better yet, a prayer (I'm hoping for a personal record, after all).

The Italians we pass as we run are absorbed in their Sunday morning routines, casually strolling, shopping, and going about their business, only occasionally stopping to look and half-heartedly clap or quietly offer *brava*. I laugh out loud when a couple and an elderly woman try to cross the street through throngs of runners— barking what must be Italian cuss words with their hands gesturing in all directions—because nobody is stopping for them. The

Italian language is so beautiful though, even the most abusive words sound like opera to my ears.

I look around and wonder, *Is it just me or are ALL Italians extraordinarily gorgeous?* People-watching in this race has reduced me to a junior-high-school girl who can't shake that ridiculous "ga-ga" look off her face. Packs of tall, dark, handsome men zoom by in racing-team formation and my eyes follow their backsides. *Dear Lord, get me to mile seventeen where my handsome hunk of a husband is waiting with refreshments. I'm looking at Italian butts, and I'm on my honeymoon, for God's sake!* I hope the pope doesn't catch onto this one.

The charm of this race is undeniable as we run through narrow cobblestone alleyways lined with warm ochre and terracotta buildings. Rainbow-colored *PACE* (peace) banners adorn windows and balconies as Italians gently voice their opposition to the Iraqi war, while classic old Fiats and scooters vie for parking spaces on neighborhood sidewalks.

After crossing the river again and looping around the northern part of the city, we head back toward the center where we run through Piazza Navona. It is here that Rome completely wraps its arms around me. I remember reading in a guidebook that this is considered one of the most beautiful baroque sites in all of Rome, but it's the vibe that captures me—people lingering at sidewalk cafes, laughing and tossing that hypnotic language back and forth to each other, not a care in the world. Of course, like all the other tourists, I'm wowed by the many classic fountains and statues, but it's "Italians doing what Italians do best" that I'm taken by most. I admire their ability to enjoy just *being*, rather than always feeling like they should be *doing* something, and I hope it rubs off on me, but right now I am busy *doing* this marathon!

I know one thing for sure: when the race is over I want to come back here and linger like an Italian over an espresso—well, no— let's make that a bottle of wine. And I want to eat thin-crust Italian pizza until I can't move, and finish it off with a gallon of gelato. It's *amoré*, just like in the Dean Martin song. His swooning voice starts wafting through my head. . . . Pllleeeeeease!

The Spanish Steps are next on our racing tour of the city. Because this is one of the most exclusive areas in Rome, drawing droves of tourists and Romans to shop in its upscale boutiques, the course is crowded here. Tourists cheer fanatically while sleek, perennially tanned Italian women in high heels saunter with shopping bags in one hand and cell phones in the other.

Just down the road we circle around the Trevi Fountain where again, throngs of tourists pack the course. This time, "Three Coins in the Fountain" serenades me as I run past the giant statue of Neptune presiding over the water below. Tradition has it that if you turn your back to the fountain and toss a coin in over your right shoulder you will one day return to Rome. I make a mental note to come back to make my offering because I already know I want to return. There's no stopping now though.

Though I've vowed to stop logging monuments in my head during this race, I can't help but take note when we pass the Pantheon, the best-preserved ancient building in Rome. I'm dying to stop in and see its famous dome and oculus, but at the moment, finishing the race is more important.

Even though I'm enjoying the charm of running through the

city on miles of cobblestones, my ankles and legs are relieved when
we reach smooth roads again. Circus Maximus, a large field where
imperial chariot races once took place, now sprawls out to our right.
It's late in the race and I'm starting to tire. There aren't many Italian butts to distract me at the moment, so I start daydreaming. I see
shades of *Ben-Hur* and picture the pomp and ceremony of the races
as emperors and aristocrats cheer from above on Palatine Hill.

Only the modest cheer of a spectator lining the course brings
me back to the present. I leave Julius Caesar's heirs behind and
focus on the task at hand: finishing this race. With only ten kilometers left, and the prospect of finishing at the Coliseum, my spirits are high.

It's the final stretch and I'm ready to wrap up my tour. But here
we go again, those clever Romans—throwing in an *uphill* push to
the finish, just for laughs. My loopy mind saves me from focusing
on my burning legs and sends me straight into the Coliseum
where I picture gladiators and animals duking it out in this
ancient amphitheater. I'm able to finish in time to run a PR, too!

As I cross the finish line, I try to digest all that I've seen on my
Roman Holiday. So much history, so much beauty, so much
humor. I can think of no better way to have experienced it,
although my tired dogs tell me that for the rest of my stay, I might
want to motor around on a scooter with my husband, the Audrey
Hepburn–way.

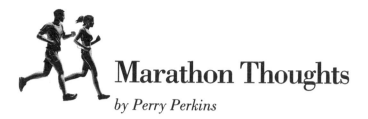

Marathon Thoughts

by Perry Perkins

Portland Marathon. October 9, 2005

- 26.2 miles is a long way. *A long way.* Way longer than our twenty-mile practice walk, infinitely longer than the ten-mile run from work to home.

- 26.2 miles is an odyssey of conflicting thoughts and emotions. Grinding, thudding pain, and hysterical laughter. It's joy at the miles behind you, despair at the ones still ahead.

- Miles one to five are euphoria. It's the crowd jostling for position, the starting gun, and the cheer of 13,000 people roaring down a skyscrapered canyon and washing over you in the semidarkness. It's the one-man rally squad at the first turn who I wish would come to the Xerox parking lot every morning and cheer me from my car to into work. "You look great man, you're doing awesome! I'm proud of you!" It's passing through the gauntlet line of cheerleaders, each of them posing for the camera. (I've waited twenty freakin' years to hear a dozen high school cheerleaders screaming my name from the sidelines; it was worth every penny and every step!)

- Miles five to ten: It's tossing your sweatshirt aside to join a thousand (ten thousand?) jackets strewn along the sidewalk like dead leaves fallen from a forest of Walmart trees. It's trying not to look ashamed that you are only walking, instead of running; from then on it's just hoping you can keep walking to the end. I mean, it's just walking, right? Good Lord, how hard can it be to just keep putting one foot in front of the other? Toddlers can do it! You're not even carrying a backpack! People do twenty-five miles a day on the Pacific Crest Trail for five *months*! What kind of a wuss is depressed at the sight of a long slow upgrade after just fifteen miles of *walking*?

- Mile eleven is retaping your feet as the first blisters start to appear. It's joking with your friends about whose stupid idea *was* this? It's cheering the sweaty, oblivious runners who are passing you coming back, and your heart breaking for the woman struggling at the very end of the walking pack, a police-escort car and a long line of traffic following her at a crawl. You can hear the revolving lights of the cruiser whispering "loser . . . loser . . . loser . . ." as she hobbles along. It's cringing and looking away.

- Mile thirteen is just unfair. After that gut-busting climb up to the bridge you discover that it's the slow walk down the other side that really hurts. It is unjust.

- Mile fifteen is the memory of six hours of nasty-tasting power bars, stomach-turning glucose drinks, and some horribly sweet sludge called Honey Stinger. It's reminding yourself to post a warning on your blog: if you ever decide to slurp down a packet of Honey Stinger, don't ever wash it down with two Red Bull energy drinks. Ever.

- Mile eighteen is the best rendition of "Free Bird" you have ever heard, or maybe you're just low on glucose again. You don't care.

- Mile twenty is realizing that the cheering and support seemed nice at first, even a little embarrassing, but now it has gone from cute, to greatly appreciated, to producing eye-watering gratefulness.

- Mile twenty-two is abandoning your friends to fate and pushing through in a heavy-metal cocoon, oblivious to cheerleaders, traffic lights (almost ending the whole walk there). It's dodging crowds of freaks at the Saturday market and leaping over sleeping bums. You let nothing slow you down now.

- Mile twenty-six is adjusting your headphones, cranking up your MP3 player so "You Shook Me All Night Long" is blaring in both ears as you walk the last 100 feet. You are finishing up between two larger groups and walk the center line down the last two blocks completely alone. It's your wife screaming "That's my husband!" just loud enough for you to hear over the music. It's knowing that nothing is better than that.

- The Finish Line. It's forgetting to check your time (who cares, you finished!). It's a bag of bananas and peanut butter cookies, a rose, and a gold medal, and strangers patting your back. It's suddenly realizing that next year's marathon will be much easier just knowing how the finish line is; what the finish line is. It's suddenly realizing that there will be a marathon next year.

- You cross the finish line totally spent, physically and emotionally exhausted, which is just how you wanted to end it.

It is a long, hard walk, but the last sixty seconds made it all worth it. Crossing the line is like a shot of speed; suddenly you no longer register the pain in your feet, the grinding of your hips. You feel great. You are a gladiator walking into the Coliseum, and all the crowds of Rome are lining the fence chanting your name, cheering. It's the post-marathon rush of endorphins that lasts about fifteen minutes. Then, as your friends cross the line (and now you feel like a dog for abandoning them earlier), you cheer with the crowd, and your feet wake back up and the glory of the finish line is overwhelmed by visions of beer, pizza, and a soft couch.

- It's your post-marathon party: crashed at your friends' house, the three of you semicomatose on a combination of Guinness, Advil, and pepperoni with extra cheese, while your wife (who is a gift from God, wonderful beyond words) plays Florence Nightingale, running more beer and pizza between foot massages.
- It's limping proudly through the office the following morning wearing your bright blue finisher's shirt and trying not to grin.
- Or maybe it's none of that for you. Maybe it's something completely different and just as completely wonderful. Maybe it's not wonderful at all.
- Maybe it's just me.

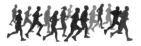

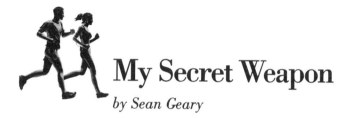

My Secret Weapon

by Sean Geary

In May 2005 I signed up to run the 25K event at the Fifth Third River Bank Run in Grand Rapids, Michigan. At about 15.5 miles, it was going to be the longest distance I had ever run, as I had skipped the three long runs in my training program that came close to that distance. However, I was undaunted. I had a secret weapon: GU Energy Gel. Mind you, I had never taken this magical substance before, but I'd heard from other runners that it gave you massive amounts of energy and kept you running for hours. So I felt there was no reason to slog twelve, thirteen, or fifteen miles through the rain and cool weather of a Michigan spring (as my official River Bank Run training program called for) when I could get the same benefits by sucking down a packet of maltodextrin. The word maltodextrin just sounds like something a skinny, superfast, elite-type runner would use.

The day before the race, I stayed with my parents who didn't live that far from the racecourse. I was nervous, but I couldn't let myself show it. My mom kept asking me if I was *sure* that I wanted to run it. After all, it was a *really long* distance. It did not seem like a long distance in February when I had the genius idea to sign up for it over beers and boasting with my best friend. The same friend who all of a sudden *had* to go to the wedding of a cousin—a wedding that just happened to be the same weekend as the race. He merely shrugged when I mentioned the fact that this cousin was so far removed from his family that he could have *married* her in most states. All of a sudden, creeping doubts planted themselves in my brain. My wife was staying at a family cottage on Lake Michigan, about an hour away, and it would have been so easy to jump in the car and curl up under the old down comforter with her.

Race morning came faster than I thought it would, especially since I decided to carbo-load the night before with my brother and Samuel Adams. The morning temperature was forty-three degrees with a light rain. After a quick bowl of Cocoa Puffs and peanut butter toast (my mother was under the impression I was thirteen, forgetting I was actually thirty), I jumped into the car with my father to head downtown.

I told my father I was shooting for a finishing time of 1:59. This lofty goal would qualify me as an elite-level runner and secure a front-of-the-pack starting place for the 2006 race. He looked at me and asked if I knew how fast I would need to run each mile. One of the lawyers in my father's firm was also running the race (she had just run the Boston Marathon the month before) and was impressed with my goal time, but warned that one would need to run sub-8-minute miles to cross the finish line in under two hours. Math was never my strong suit, which my father knew, and neither was distance running. Put the two together and we had a pending disaster. Still, I was undaunted because GU would give me the speed and stamina to finish in my goal time, but also leave me with enough energy to laugh heartily at all those who doubted my delusions of grandeur.

I moseyed up to the starting line and milled around with the pace group for eight-minute miles. Not too far ahead I could see the sign that read UNDER TWO HOURS, directing runners with a similar goal to mine. The rain started to pick up a bit as the national anthem was played and the wheelchair racers were sent out. My liquid courage from the night before was gurgling in my belly and I was not exactly "cuckoo" for the Cocoa Puffs that I ingested for breakfast. I was also regretting the shorts I had chosen to wear instead of running tights. The thin material had long since lost the wicking battle with the incessant rain and was now cold and clinging to my pasty legs. Before I had time to pick the liner out of my nether-regions, my group was pressing toward the front. People were shouting and jumping and pushing forward and then *stopping*! I ran right up the back of the fellow in front of me—the masses slowed at the starting mat to start their watches. We were not off to an auspicious start.

Before too long an audible beep came from the timing chips on our shoes, signaling and recording our start, and we were running. I tried to pay attention to the buildings we passed downtown as we ran, and I let my mind fall back to my high school days in the city. I remember checking my new running watch every fifteen seconds, wondering how far we had run. The rain was cold and annoying and it was hard to find room to run at any sort of even pace in the crush of humanity around me. Finally the first mile came and went, and we thinned out a bit. My first mile was a second or two over eight minutes. I was right on target.

I saw the aid station at mile two and moved to my left, away from the largest of the groups of people moving to the water and sports drinks on the right. I skipped the first table and looked to the second when I saw a volunteer holding up a surgically gloved hand that was covered in a glistening, viscous substance.

Could this be the GU I had heard so much about? I was confused. I thought it might be a little early in the course to offer GU, but what did I know? I convinced myself that it would not be too early. If the race lasted two to three hours, you would want some energy gel in the first part of the race and somewhere in the middle to take you over the finish line, right? I knew there were two stations for GU, so why not here?

I made a beeline for the volunteer, even pointing at her so she knew that the hulking, soaking, stinking mass headed in her direction was doing so *with a purpose*. I wanted her GU. She smiled (probably stifling a laugh) and stuck her hand out. I slapped it hard and dragged my hand across hers, not wanting to waste any of the precious substance that hung there completely unaffected by gravity and seemingly put there by the good Lord Himself.

I looked at the substance that now coated my left hand in awe and amazement. This stuff was going to give my ankles wings and carry me across the finish line with no problems. My, how foolish my detractors would look! I brought my hand to my mouth and a little part of my brain registered the strange fact that GU *repelled water*. Seriously, the rain was beading up on it and flying right off. Could that be right?

I expelled the doubts from my brain; after all, who was I to argue with the greatest scientific dietary achievement since Tang? I shoved my fingers into my mouth and scrapped them clean. Or as clean as I could get—that stuff was sticky! I could not get it all off. I licked and sucked as I ran. It tasted a lot different than I thought it would, not at all like the "plain" taste advertised in the brochure. I did not gag or toss it up, so it was not all that bad.

Before I knew it, my legs were churning faster and my speed was increasing! I felt *great*! My stomach was settled—no more gross beer burps—and I felt like I could go forever! I was two and a half miles into the run and I felt like I was walking, except I was running, and fast. By mile three, I was below a 7:50 pace and right on track for breaking two hours. This stuff was like legalized *cheating*!

Mile 4.5 brought the next aid station and I went to the left again. The rain was letting up a bit, but it was still much colder than I would have liked, since I was soaking wet and wearing shorts. I spotted volunteers holding crushed (so they were easier to drink) cups of water and Gatorade and then I spotted another volunteer with the gloved hand outstretched. *What?* Both GU stations in the first five miles? How was I supposed to end my suffering at mile ten? Did they expect me to carry the stuff with me for the next hour or so? *Maybe*, I thought, *this was for people who were not ready for it at the last station, but now they would be.* I convinced myself that this made sense.

As I got closer I realized the volunteer was holding her right hand (with the surgical glove) out with the same viscous, gravity-defying goop on it and holding a tub in her left hand. The tub looked familiar. It was industrial size and had a familiar yellowish tint with a blue cap. Where had I seen that before? Suddenly my brain locked in on it. I knew exactly where I had seen that stuff before. *In my medicine cabinet at home.* My mind reeled in utter horror as the weight of my actions descended on me like a piano.

I HAD JUST EATEN VASELINE.

What was wrong with me? How could I have been so naïve? My stupidity was astounding. Where was my common sense? Why would volunteers serve GU *off their hands?* Who thinks like that? Wouldn't GU come in little packets? No wonder it repelled water and would not come off my fingers. *That was its job!* It was petroleum jelly, not maltodextrin! Horror rose up from the animal portion of my brain, the part that told early man to stay away from things like saber-tooth tigers, funny mushrooms, and fruit. *You were not supposed to eat that stuff!*

I looked around. I was surrounded by hundreds of cold, wet, sweaty, panting runners. *How many of them watched me eat Vaseline?* When we all crossed the finish line (under two hours) and were standing around eating bagels and basking in the glow of elitism, would I overhear one guy saying to another, "You know, craziest thing happened. I was running next to this guy and he takes a big handful of Vaseline from a volunteer *and eats it!* Who *does* that?"

Would I become a joke to the very people I was trying to emulate? How would they explain it to my wife when she had to identify me at the hospital? "Sorry ma'am, it looks like he ingested a lethal amount of petroleum jelly. Probably in the form of over-the-counter lubricant like Vaseline. Do you have any idea why he would do that? Did he have mental problems or very poor eyesight? Who eats *Vaseline?*"

Things could not get any worse. And then my iPod died.

It had soaked up too much water and shorted out *in the middle of an awesome song.* Was I really going to have to run the next ten miles with Audioslave's "Like a Stone" in my head? I hardly knew any lyrics other than the chorus! I knew that if the Vaseline did not kill me, I would wish that it did after forty minutes of repeating the same line over and over again in my head.

What I failed to realize at the time was I was still running *fast.* No drop in stamina, no pain, just one foot in front of the other. Mile six came and went and then mile seven and *real* GU.

How did mile seven get here so fast? I thought. No time to contemplate space-time continuum; I would wait on that until I had an opportunity to try LSD. Instead, I grabbed my packet of GU Chocolate Outrage and an orange Gatorade and continued to run along. I ripped open the package of GU, took a sniff, and finding it rather unrevolting, I shoved it in my mouth and squeezed.

Having no idea what to expect, I was pleasantly surprised when it hit my tongue. It tasted like brownie batter. I washed it down with the Gatorade and kept on going. Let me say this now: nothing says delicious like orange Gatorade and Chocolate Outrage. Yuck.

The rain kept up, the course got hilly, and my times dropped ever so slightly; 7:50s became 8:14s, and I found that I no longer cared about my finishing time. Mile ten came and went and then we were in sight of the city again at mile twelve. All of a sudden, my iPod started up again. Everything is going to be *great!*

Until my quads started that slow burn and I could feel my breaths getting shorter. Another aid station and another packet of GU. I reached out my hand for the life-giving substance, giving the Vaseline Volunteer a wide berth, and got a packet of . . .

berry??? What? I hate fruit. I *loathe* fruit. Nothing could be worse. What happened to everything going so great???

Blessings come in small packages, even ones with fruit inside them. I did not eat this package but stared at it, filled with despair and rage. *How could this happen to me? What did I do to deserve this?* I ranted and raved in my head and I kept running. My mind was so focused on the cosmic insult of berry GU that I forgot completely about the pain in my legs, and I just ran. Mile thirteen came and went. I cannot even remember mile fourteen to this day. Next thing I knew we were running next to Grand Valley State University's downtown campus and we were just about a mile from the end. *Could this really be happening?*

I remember very clearly that the next song that came on my iPod was "Last Train Home" by the Lostprophets. This was my favorite song at the time, and it has the perfect beat to run *fast.* I tossed the packet to the side of the road and just ran. We went up and over the river next to the Gerald R. Ford Museum and the finish line got closer and closer. I forgot completely about the watch and just kept my legs moving. My lungs were on fire and my breath was coming in short rasps. My heart rate monitor indicated I was over 180 beats per minute. I was a freight train.

I was unstoppable, but no one told me about the incline for the last quarter mile. I was convinced that there was no oxygen left in the atmosphere, only fire and glass. My lungs ached; my tongue was dry and thick. My knees hurt with every pounding step. I could no longer hear the music in my headphones because of the blood pounding in my ears up to my brain. How long is a quarter mile? One thousand three-hundred and twenty never-ending feet of torture, pain, despair, and triumph.

I crossed the line. The announcer said my name and number. I slowed down, my legs shaking, my eyes blurry from sweat and rainwater. A volunteer helped me untie the timing chip from my shoe (only after I noticed that he was not carrying Vaseline). I walked over toward the tents where an army of volunteers was handing out bananas, bagels, and bottles of water. My dad found me shortly after and gave me a big, disgusting hug, and I managed not to throw up on him. It was one of my prouder moments.

To this day, I still listen at the start of races to hear if anyone tells the story of the runner from the 2005 River Bank Run who ate Vaseline, but I have yet to hear it. The story itself has grown in legend among my circle of friends. In 2006 when my best friend ran the River Bank with me (I guess he was out of cousins to watch get married) he shouted, "Don't eat the Vaseline!" at the first aid station. Everyone looked at him like he was from the moon. I regaled most of the Coast Guard runners at the 2007 Traverse City State Bank Bayshore Marathon between miles eight and fourteen with the Vaseline story and it made the hill climb and turnaround at mile 13.1 that much more enjoyable. I wish I had waited until mile twenty-one to tell it.

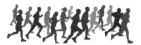

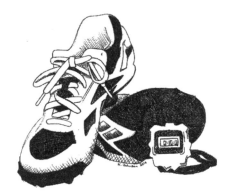

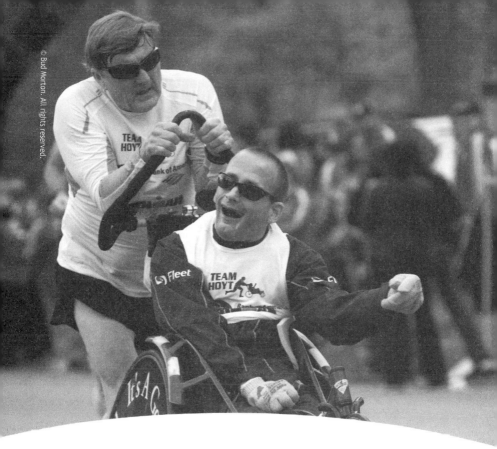

Running for
a Cause

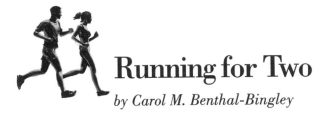

Running for Two

by Carol M. Benthal-Bingley

I f you've shared a good run with someone, you've created a bond with that person for life. We runners have a bond because we share something in common. We have a connection beyond the surface. We've seen each other at our best and our worst. We've seen each other physically and emotionally drained from pushing ourselves farther than we thought we could be pushed. We push each other, and when we fall, we pick each other up. We're part of a unique community, a family of runners with all our strengths and beautiful flaws.

I met Annie, a dear friend of my sister, about five years ago. She was a beautiful woman . . . talented, energetic, bright, vibrant, and she was a runner. I wasn't much of a runner at the time, but I wanted to be. She helped me train for and race my first triathalon. She was amazing: strong, elegant—and dying of cancer.

Last year, around the time her doctor had given her only two more months to live, I bumped into Annie. She asked me to run for her until she could run again. She shared how she'd missed running; how she missed feeling the breeze in her hair as she ran;

how she longed to go out and just run, and keep on running.

A group of us decided to run for Annie. We logged miles and miles for our "sister." We offered up the run for our friend, a woman most of the group had never met. We had a bond with her, through her, to do something outside of ourselves. To offer up that run to whomever it is we pray to. We were running for two. Running for someone else, someone who missed running desperately. We started out doing it for her, and quickly realized how much she was doing for us. She was giving us strength, inspiring us every step of the way.

Annie died a few weeks ago. This incredible woman had been given two years to live—that was six years ago. She was given six months a few years ago. Her endurance was beyond anything we could imagine. When she was given forty-eight hours, she took another week. She fought all the way to the finish line. Her body was done, but something way beyond physical strength took over. She stayed on this earth longer, running toward her own finish line, not giving in until her race was won.

A few months ago I read an article in *Runners World* written by Kristin Armstrong (Lance's ex-wife). It was about a marathon she'd run with a friend. How they'd run the miles, dedicating each mile to someone they loved. They prayed for that person for a mile then moved on to the next. I thought that was beautiful. The idea stuck with me as we ran all those months for Annie.

Last week at the Rock Cut Hobo Run 25K near Rockford, Illinois, my friend Julie and I decided to run the 15.5 mile trail race in honor of Annie. It was a beautiful day, a Sunday, a day Annie would have loved to run. We ran to the first mile marker, slapped hands, and decided to whom we'd dedicate each mile as it came. We ran for Annie, her lovely daughter, her two brave sons, her loving husband, her dear "sisters," and for Annie again. We rotated through the people whom Annie loved. It was such an emotional, spiritual journey running through those woods, gaining steam at each mile. We thought about the endurance this woman had, the strength she showed as she faced her own mortality, and the dignity and grace she wore as she fought this unimaginable battle. When we had thoughts of doubt and pain and feeling tired, we thought of Annie. We know that the small amount of endurance we exhibited that day was nothing compared to the race Annie had just completed.

By mile eight, I was tired. When the next mile marker came up, Julie and I regrouped, slapped hands, and said "This one's for Annie." I started off on the second half of the Hobo Run, winding through the trees, the sun spilling through the leaves. I closed my eyes for a second, consciously breathing in the fresh air. Just then something filled me up—I felt lighter, energized, refilled. I cannot give credit to my sports drink or energy gels for this one. This was beyond the chemistry of complex carbs and electrolytes. I believe I felt the presence of something bigger and the warmth of knowing that Annie was smiling, and probably somewhere out there . . . running! I finished the race, worn out and filled up. I watched for Julie. She came cruising in with an amazing energy and a decisive surge at the finish. We were exhausted and energized, laughing and crying. She shared how she'd pooped out the last mile and a half, thinking she wouldn't finish.

She said she'd just flown in on Annie's wings.

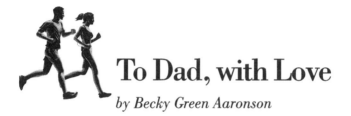

To Dad, with Love

by Becky Green Aaronson

It's 6:00 AM and my alarm mercifully rescues me from an endless night of tossing and turning. As I lay in a sleep-deprived daze, I stare into the darkness of my hotel room and try to imagine what the next ten hours will bring. I've been training for this day for nearly a year and dreaming about it since I was a teenager, yet I can't coax myself out of bed. Instead I think about my dad, the slender, witty man I miss every day. Fourteen years ago, cancer killed him.

Soon, my back-up alarm jolts me out of my reverie, followed by a wake-up call from the front desk. As I sit on the edge of the bed, I try to focus on the task at hand, but my mind wanders back nearly twenty years to the Trails End Marathon in Seaside, Oregon. On a cold, rainy day I volunteered to hand out water to runners as they battled the course and the elements. I was only a kid, but I admired those competitors as they triumphed over the 26.2 miles. I knew then I wanted to be a marathon runner.

The memory sends a charge of excitement through me as I contemplate my challenge today: the New York City Marathon. The only thing that would make this day more perfect is if my dad was here to share it with me. In a sense, he will be.

It took many years before I decided to enter my first marathon, but it took no time at all to decide which one to run. I chose the mother of them all—New York—because it's one of the largest and craziest. I wanted this experience to be memorable, especially if it turned out to be my only marathon. I also planned to use the race to raise money for cancer research, because the disease had profoundly affected my family.

My dad, who had always seemed healthy, was diagnosed with lung cancer at age fifty-two. Even after all these years, it's hard to reconcile the reality of his disease with my memories of him. I can still picture him running me all over the tennis court for hours. Near the end, he occasionally complained about a nagging pain in his back, one he attributed to years of hard work and arthritis. What he brushed off as insignificant turned out to be cancer, a scourge that quickly spread throughout his body, taking his life just six months later.

My mom would also grapple with this disease. Though she conquered breast cancer several years ago, it wasn't without painful surgery and lengthy treatments. Watching both of my parents suffer through cancer angered and frustrated me, because I felt powerless to do anything but lend my support.

The NYC Marathon finally gave me a chance to fight back. I planned to gather pledges for every mile I ran and donate the money to a leading cancer center. When I discovered Memorial Sloan-Kettering's "Fred's Team" program (named in honor of Fred Lebow, the former director of the NYC Marathon who died of cancer), I signed up and poured my heart into fund-raising. In the end, it became almost more important to me than running the marathon itself.

On race morning my enthusiasm is reinforced as I pull on my orange-and-purple Fred's Team uniform. Wearing the uniform makes it all seem real for the first time. Then I stretch slowly as my husband, Jeffrey, offers words of encouragement.

Finally we head out the door and down Central Park South to Mickey Mantle's Restaurant where Sloan-Kettering is hosting a prerace bagel party for Fred's Team. The unfamiliar faces there do nothing to calm my nerves. My teammates welcome me warmly, though, and I begin to relax as we take pictures and board our celebrity VIP limousines.

At first I don't fully understand the significance of our "celebrity" status, but it becomes clear as sirens wail and lights flash; we're being led through the streets of New York by a police escort. People along the way try to figure out who we are, likely thinking we're the elite runners. It makes us giddy. We laugh and cheer as officers stop traffic to wave us through.

On Staten Island we join the other runners inside Fort Wadsworth, which has been transformed into an athletes' village. I wade through the sea of humanity and see every kind of person wearing every kind of outfit. I also hear the buzz of many different languages. Funny characters abound; I can only imagine the classic one-liners Dad would have had about them. He'd get a kick out of the runner sporting a rhino costume and the grandfather wearing a shirt made entirely of bib numbers from previous NYC Marathons.

Before the race I seek out a restroom but discover the lines are a mile long. Even hundreds of Porta-Johns aren't enough for 30,000 runners. I join the line and pass the time chatting with people, including a New Yorker in his midforties who's running his tenth NYC Marathon. He's thrilled that I'm running my first and says, "It's something you will *never* forget. It's right up there with getting married and having children—*major* life events." I also talk with a Scottish man, a member of a large group from Edinburgh, running to raise money for cancer research. Knowing others around the world are trying to tackle this disease makes me want to hug him.

I finally get my turn in the Porta-John, then hustle to the starting area on the Verrazano-Narrows Bridge. Helicopters hover overhead and my heart races with adrenaline. I borrow a marker from someone and write "DAD" prominently on my hand to reinforce the significance of this day. Although nobody knows I'm running this race in honor of Dad, I have a feeling *he* knows, and that's all that matters. At 10:45 AM, the national anthem reverberates, then a few minutes later Mayor Giuliani fires the cannon. We're off!

For the first nine miles I'm running on clouds, carried by the spectators, costumes, bands, and signs lining the route. As I pass a Nike billboard with the slogan, "5 Boroughs, 26.2 miles, and 29,000 dreams," my thoughts turn to those around me. I wonder why each person is running this marathon. I'm sure every answer is different.

My own reason for running gives me a deeply rooted sense of strength and hope. I know my contribution to cancer research is a drop in the bucket, but I feel empowered knowing that I'm doing *something* about the disease that shattered my family. I hope Mom's recent brush with cancer will be her last. At that moment a spectator yells, "Good job, Fred's Team!"

The next six miles are filled with nonstop support and entertainment. I realize I haven't stopped smiling for over two hours. That is until I reach the 59th Street Bridge, which is long, and devoid of spectators. I'm left with nothing to focus on but my knotted quads, and I'm convinced this bridge will go on forever.

To stay inspired and distract myself long enough to get over the bridge, I start thinking of the people who sponsored me: Janet, Sarah, Bill, Mom. If I get to mile sixteen, I'll have raised more than $3,300 for research. If I reach the end, it will be much more. I have to keep going. Margie, Elizabeth, Mark, Donna. My tactic works. Soon I see the end of the bridge and hear the roar of the crowd. I'm re-energized.

Not only do I make it over the bridge but I manage to reach mile eighteen before I finally stop and stretch. As I do, I look at my hand—the one marked "DAD"—and ask him to help me make it through the rest of the race. Soon I'm on my way again, enjoying it more than I ever imagined.

In Harlem, a woman hollers, "Oh Baby, you're lookin' so good, you're lookin' so strong, you just keep on going! You are a winner, you hear me? You are a *winner!*" I want to hug her, too, but my legs tell me I can't stop now.

At mile twenty-two, it finally hits me: I'm going to make it! After a year of training and months of fund-raising, I'm almost there. The closer I get, the prouder I feel. As I cross the finish line in Central Park, I'm euphoric. With a lump in my throat, I say quietly, "Dad, I hope you're proud. This was for you."

Afterward, I receive a rose and a finisher's medal, then I'm wrapped in a colorful Mylar blanket and escorted to the special Fred's Team area where friends and family are gathered. Never before have I felt so tired—and so alive.

As Jeffrey and I make our way back to the hotel, which seems miles away, I garner nods of approval from complete strangers. I remember giving that same nod to the runners I so admired almost twenty years ago. I also feel the warmth of my dad's smile. I know we'll be running together again next year.

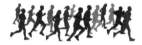

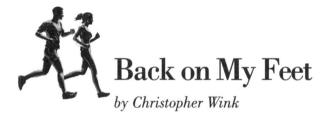

Back on My Feet

by Christopher Wink

Matthew used to break a lot of promises. He'd lie to girl-friends about why he needed money and why he didn't pay them back. He'd tell someone he would do something or be somewhere without much intention of ever following through. He'd disappear, stay out for a few nights, and return home with some bogus excuse. He used drugs and sold drugs. He smoked and drank.

Matthew also used to be a runner. In high school and college, he was a sprinter. He was fast.

At some point he stopped running for two decades. Long enough to walk a path few return from, but Matthew did, running all the way back.

In 2007, Anne Mahlum would take long, solitary runs in the early morning twilight of Center City Philadelphia. Every day, she'd run a particular route that would bring her past a group of residents outside a mission. Soon they began to wave to each other and exchange hellos; later they'd share small greetings and the relationship grew.

After one run, she had a moment of clarity.

"I just stopped and looked behind me and thought, 'What am I doing?'" Anne said. "I started to realize, 'I'm moving my life forward every day, physically, emotionally, mentally, and these guys are standing in the same spot.'"

So that July, Anne decided that a great way to combat homelessness in Philadelphia was to give out pairs of sneakers and get a running club together with her new friends. The North Dakota native and avid runner was due to start a high-paying job with a Fortune 100 company, and thought she might start the program and work on it in her free time.

It was about confidence and community building, goals and structure, and the sense of an accomplishment after feet hit pavement. Soon, she'd bring on job development and training partners, but from the first mile, Back on My Feet was always about the running.

In the first few weeks of soliciting donations for running gear and getting more guys from the mission involved, a funny thing happened. Anne got a taste of the power of the idea she was developing. Running developed relationships fast, and the potential loomed large.

The night before she was due in for her first day at her new job, Anne called her soon-to-be boss and announced she wouldn't be coming in. She'd found a new direction.

"When you're part of witnessing someone discovering their potential and everything they're capable of, there's nothing better," Anne said. "It's like I found my purpose, why I'm here, and you can't pick these moments. They just happen."

Born in Frankfurt, Germany, in 1968 to a U.S. Army family,

Matthew lived in Virginia and Texas but grew up mostly in a fraying Philadelphia neighborhood of the 1980s.

"I was a good kid but easily misled by guys I thought were good friends," Matthew says. By the time he was fifteen, he was drinking regularly; by eighteen, he'd found weed, and after graduating high school, he was introduced to cocaine. He worked construction but always dealt and used and partied. What started as a kid having fun became a man with a problem.

"It's the same old story. I thought I was cool, but I lost control at some point," he said.

The same month in the same city that Anne launched her program to run with homeless populations, Matthew had his moment of sanity and moved into a shelter. "I just realized that I had wasted my last twenty years," Matthew said. "Everything became clear, and I decided that I wanted my life back."

From getting tossed out of college for fighting and tossed into jail for drug possession offenses, to the drinking and the dealing and, yes, the lying, Matthew needed a new way. Two days later he was in a treatment program. A month later, he moved to a rehabilitation facility, where he could focus on staying clean but get home to help his girlfriend with his two kids and her three.

"I was always supposed to be taking care of them," Matthew said. "But it wasn't until then that I ever really did."

By September 2007, Back on My Feet had added a team at a second facility and was looking for a third. The next month, Anne easily found another partner and addressed the facility's residents, Matthew among them, about her program and the direction they were headed toward, offering help beyond running instruction.

"I can remember thinking 'here she is, this little white lady try-ing to save the world.' I laughed. I didn't think it was serious. It was a joke," Matthew said. "It was just something to do." Matthew joined and soon found the backbone of Back on My Feet.

He had to wake up at 5:00 AM and be outside ready to run at 5:30 AM every Monday, Wednesday, and Friday. He'd get sneak-ers and some running gear, but only if he kept up the program's mandatory 90 percent attendance. His miles would be tracked. He'd get job interviews, life-skills training and support, but only if he ran farther and faster. "There isn't anything easy about Back on My Feet. Looking back, the concept is too perfect, getting people back on their feet," Matthew said. "After a few runs, it began to make a difference in my life because I wasn't alone. There was a team; you make friends and remember how to trust again."

At each facility, volunteers and other members form a com-munity. "The support from the volunteers is still inspiring. You never ran alone and there was always conversation," Matthew said. "I worked hard to be able to be in good enough shape to talk while I ran so I could stay in the conversation."

The Back on My Feet conversations continue today in Balti-more, Washington, D.C., and Boston, with plans to expand to other cities. The conversations always vary, but running doesn't ever seem to be far from the topic at hand. It becomes a bonding experience. Middle-aged businessmen and college athletes and teenagers and mothers become the friends and supporters of a diverse array of men and women who want to change the direc-tion of their lives. Often the goals toward making that change come in a runner's increment.

"I cried when I ran five miles for the first time," Matthew said. "That was the longest I ever ran. It was a goal, a commitment that I made, no excuses or false promises or any of the lies that I had done for years. For so long I would promise to do something and never would do it. Finally, I did something I said I would do. I don't know if I ever felt that sense of accomplishment before. That brought me to the trail that I am on now."

Back on My Feet helped Matthew get a job interview, helped him with what to say and what to wear. He nabbed steady custodial work at a regional university. Every morning, he'd run three or five miles, then dash back to the facility where he was staying to shower and change before rushing off to work with the "most energy I had ever had."

Today, Matthew is a thick guy, six-foot-three with a thin goatee, caramel-black skin, and cleanly shaved head. He has years of sobriety behind him. He's always loved to smile but says Back on My Feet helped make that a little easier.

"When you show people trust, and opportunity and love and support, that's going to stir up positive emotions and positive choices for them because they're going to realize how great life is when you make those good decisions," Anne said.

"I told her once, 'Anne, this thing is going to be bigger than you ever imagined.' She just laughed," Matthew said. "But I think I'm right."

He's living with his new fianceé, doting over a new child, and climbing the ranks of the custodial department of a local university, where he's held steady work since 2007. "I had to go through what I put myself through to love life in the way I do, and Back on My Feet played such a large role in getting me where I am now," Matthew said. "Life is beautiful, even on a rainy and cloudy day, because I know now that the sun will eventually shine, and you can always go for a run, no matter the weather."

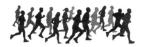

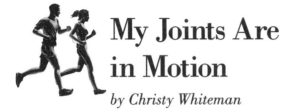

My Joints Are
in Motion

by Christy Whiteman

W hat would possess anyone to run for hours and hours
with absolutely no chance of winning and little to
show for it but a medal and a very sore body? Why would anyone
subject herself to this level of pain? Sometimes you just need a
little motivation.

More than one year ago, we found ourselves with a busy two-
year-old daughter who climbed and jumped and ran like most
other children do. Occasionally, though, she limped and she
seemed to have a strange run. We thought little of it, until one
day she refused to walk and began to cry uncontrollably. What
we thought might have been a sprained ankle or torn ligament
turned out to be something much more.

Our daughter, Reese, was diagnosed with juvenile rheumatoid
arthritis. We learned she had a type that could not be outgrown,
but could have periods of remission with the right course of treatments. In the meantime, the damage to her legs, elbows, and
hands must be immediately corrected, followed by physiotherapy,
injectable medications, and lifestyle adjustments. We had visions
of a life less fulfilled for a child not yet three years old. Since then,

we have learned to live with it and while we have no idea what will happen in the future, we feel that she is getting the best care possible.

My husband and I are not scientists or doctors, but we wanted to do something positive to help Reese and others, so we did what we knew—we registered with the Arthritis Society of Canada and I joined the Joints in Motion Training Team. Thanks to the enormous generosity of our friends and family we raised over $6,500 in just a few months and so my training to run a marathon began!

I would love to tell you that I followed the training schedule to the letter, but kids, work, husband, house, Mother Nature, family—life—got in the way a few times. I had fantastic support, not only from my family and friends, but even from those who thought I was insane for attempting the marathon. I have always been athletic, but this was the farthest distance I had ever attempted to run.

I trained in heat, rain, snow, rain, more snow, arctic winds, and the occasional blizzard. There were many, many days I wanted to bail out of the whole thing but I would usually get a supportive boost from my husband. He would spout out all the accomplishments I had reached to date. When I shared my doubts with my friends, they would flood me with "This too shall pass" comments. And so it did. In January, I left Toronto with my husband, my two children, and my parents. We were destined for Florida with more than 100 members of the Joints in Motion Training Team who would join more than 40,000 participants in the Walt Disney World Marathon weekend.

To say that the experience was magical would be an understatement. I was of two minds going into this, my first marathon. Part of me wanted to train hard and run a stellar race in a respectable finish time. The other part of me wanted the family to have a fantastic vacation and relish watching my children experience the magic of Disney for the first time. Running the marathon would be an added bonus! In the end, I took the second approach. There are few circumstances where one would parade around gigantic amusement parks in the days coming into a marathon, but I loved every second of it. My children were three and six years old, and to see them enjoy themselves was spectacular. I would not have changed a thing about my decision.

With marathon morning upon us, I was extremely nervous but also excited that this long-awaited goal would finally be attained. The fireworks at the start line set us off, and I felt great . . . for about fifteen miles. The wonderful thing about the Walt Disney World Marathon is running through several parks. What other marathon runs you through Cinderella's Castle? I saw fabulous costumes and catchy T-shirts, tiara-adorned sprinters and fairy-winged joggers. Somewhere around mile eighteen I saw a wedding proposal! I chatted with people from all over North America and a few who lived less than five miles from my house. I soaked up the energy from the extraordinary spectators, and I anticipated seeing my entire family at the finish line when it was over.

If there was a way I could have jumped ship with some dignity at mile twenty I would have done it. However, I couldn't bring myself to admit defeat, nor could I bear the thought of the faces of my family and the hundreds of others who had donated to my cause. I met a woman with the same feelings who was kind enough to lend me her cell phone to call my family. She and I became best friends for the last 6.2 miles. As I approached mile twenty-five, I still hadn't seen any of my family and I was a wreck. I was well beyond exhausted, in a lot of pain, and I wanted this race to end more than can be put into words. But at mile twenty-six, there they were. That was enough to finish 0.2 miles and cross that finish line with arms up—picture ready!

Through the corrals I kept talking to myself and became giddy with excitement over my Mickey Mouse medal! I found teammates and was met with bear hugs and handshakes. I looked like I had just been running for nearly six hours. When I finally met up with my family, my tears flowed all over again! While many of the men had flowers for women crossing the line, my husband had brought me a mint-chocolate chip ice cream cone, which was far superior and likely the envy of all those around me holding useless bouquets!

The great thing about running a marathon at Disney is that you wear your medal all around the parks for the few days after the race and as a result, you are met with agreeable nods from fellow participants, cheers from employees, and kind words from strangers. One attraction had everyone wearing a medal stand up (this took some time) while the entire group of 5,000 applauded. I will remember the Disney experience for a very long time and cannot recommend it enough to everyone who runs. Even if you don't run, it's a fantastic experience.

Ultimately, our goals were met. We raised a great deal of money for an organization whose research led to the development of a treatment from which my daughter has received tremendous benefit. I managed to finish a marathon, and we had a wonderful family vacation.

So when asked why I did it, my answer is simple: I ran for those who benefit from the research, and I ran for the people who participate in the programs. Many ran for someone they love, and I ran for my daughter. I ran for Reese with my whole heart. My joints were in motion because, some days, hers are not.

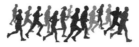

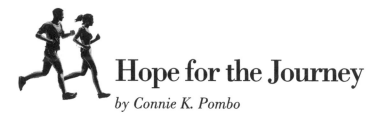

Hope for the Journey

by Connie K. Pombo

"**P**lease tell me I'm not the last runner?" I shouted. "No—keep going!" the crowd cheered back. Afraid to look over my shoulder, I continued my slow but steady pace.

I heard noisemakers and more shouts as I ran, jogged, and "crawled" my way through the first mile of the Susan G. Komen Race for the Cure. As I headed toward the first hill, a fellow runner whizzed past me with a baby jogger. She sported a pink ribbon cap, worn backwards, and her twins—a boy and a girl—wore T-shirts with the words, "In memory of Helen—wife, mother, and friend."

Tears betrayed me . . . first one . . . then two . . . until they mixed with the sweat that poured off my face. I realized for the first time that I was running—not only for me—but for every woman who ever heard the words, "You have breast cancer."

It was my first race since being diagnosed, and—of course—I ran against medical advice! As my feet dangled back and forth on the exam room table during my first post-op visit, I asked the surgeon, "So am I ready to run again?" He gave me a stern look and said, "It's only been two weeks since your surgery and I don't advise it, but you'll probably do it anyway."

He was absolutely right! I filled out my application, gathered sponsors, and entered the race the very next day. Cancer had taken away many things, but I was only forty years old, and it wasn't going to take away my running.

What my surgeon didn't know—what he possibly couldn't understand—was running saved my life. From the moment I first heard the words, "You have breast cancer," I continued with my normal running routine—three miles a day. It became a symbol of hope.

Just then, a fellow runner gave me a "high-five." She wore a pink T-shirt, pink running shoes, and pink hair that emerged from her baseball cap. As she scooted past me, she smiled and said, "Keep it up—only two miles to go!"

What? Two miles . . . no way! I thought.

Sweat continued to pour off my body while I nursed a cramped calf muscle. My lungs worked doubly hard to force the air out in small increments—two puffs at a time. I started to waver in my resolve—there was no way I was going to finish this race. *Maybe if I slipped into the crowd and walked home, no one would notice?*

As I drifted off course and wandered into the maze of spectators, I heard a voice. "Oh, no you don't!" shouted a runner behind me. She grabbed me by my pink shirttails and pulled me back into the race. *Who is this person and why is she tugging on me?* It was then I noticed her pink shirt; it read: "CANCER ISN'T FOR WIMPS!"

"Are you a quitter?" she asked.

"Yes . . . I mean . . . no! Oh, I don't know," I stammered. "I just don't think I can finish *this* race."

"Aw, sure you can," she said. "I'll run with you—okay?"

"Well, why not?" I agreed.

While she ran (and I jogged), I learned the "pink-haired lady" was a four-time cancer survivor, and this was her fifth Race for the Cure. She was twenty-four years old when she first heard the words, "You have breast cancer." And she had chemo and radiation —not once, but three times! The cancer had now spread to her bones and lungs.

As she spoke, I blinked back tears. "You look dehydrated . . . maybe you need to drink more water and do less crying," she said with a crooked smile.

The crowd cheered us on—the two breast-cancer buddies— one sporting pink hair and one wearing a pink ribbon cap. "This is my first Race for the Cure," I said. "But I didn't *know* that it was going to be this hard."

"Cancer is *just* like this race," she said defiantly. "It's all uphill with a few curves thrown in just for fun." She smacked her gum and blew a huge bubble that burst—leaving a web of pink all over her face. We giggled like schoolgirls, and then a wave of somber reality spread across her face. "Cancer is messy; you've got to learn to deal with it," she added.

If I was looking for sympathy that day, I didn't find it. My breast-cancer buddy raced ahead of me and yelled, "I'll see you at the finish line!"

Suddenly the roar of the crowd empowered me. Banners, balloons, and messages of hope carried me along as I melted into another group of runners. As I passed the second mile mark, I grabbed a cup of water that was offered to me and resolved to finish the race.

In the distance, I saw an arch of pink and white balloons that formed the finish line. It was then I caught a glimpse of my boys who were just nine and fourteen—jumping up and down—screaming, "C'mon, Mom you can do it!" I watched as my husband brushed the tears from his eyes and slid his arms around our boys.

It was then I realized *why* I was running; it was for them! I wanted our boys to remember their mom as one who ran for her life and never looked back.

It's been twelve years since I ran my first Race for the Cure (one race for every year of my life since cancer). That day, I found three reasons for running; they were waiting for me at the finish line. They were the ones who gave me hope for the journey!

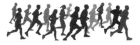

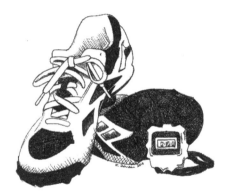

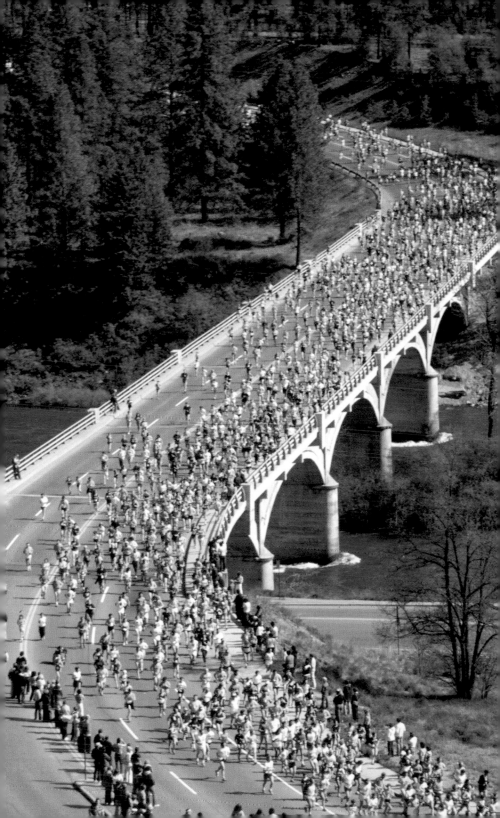

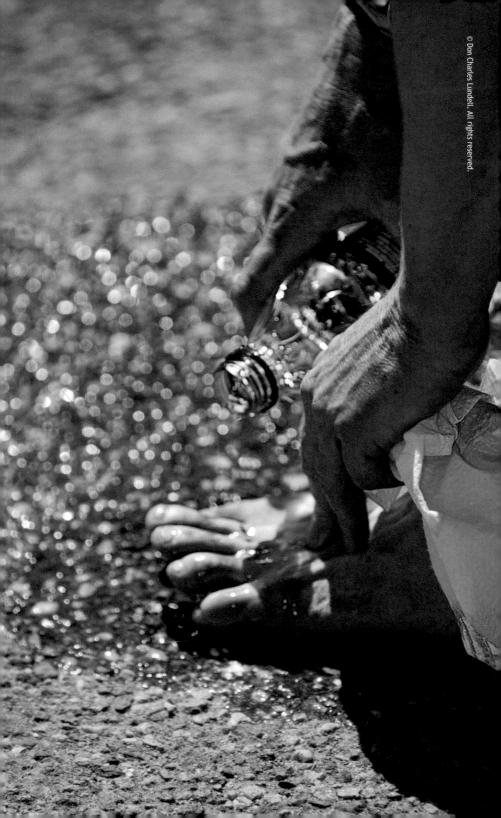

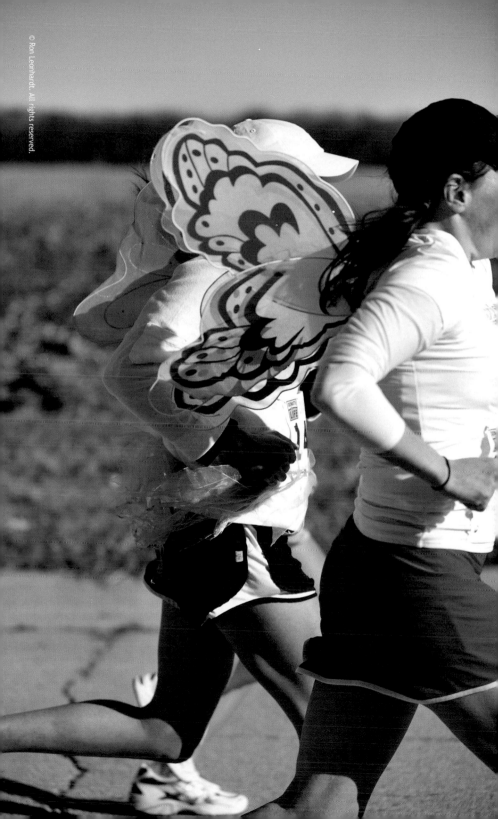

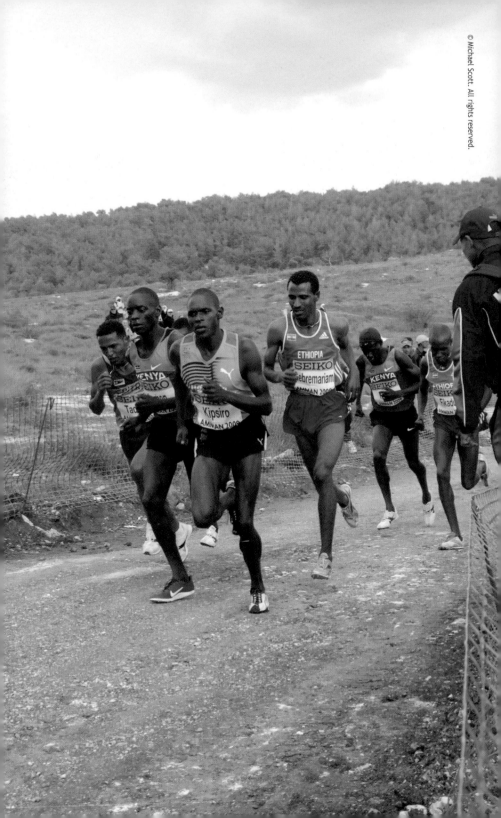

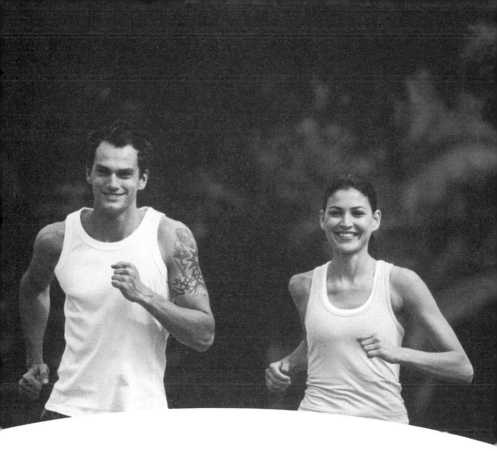

Must-Know Info

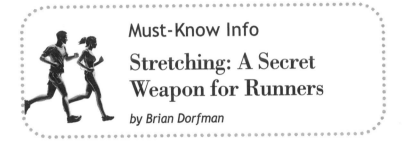

Stretching: A Secret Weapon for Runners

by Brian Dorfman

If there was a supplement that could improve recovery and circulation, promote correct biomechanics, boost performance, and prevent injuries, most of us would buy a lifetime supply. Unfortunately no such supplement exists, but a regular stretching routine can offer these same benefits in just thirty minutes. Stretching, like nutritional support, should be an integral part of your training and is the key to long-term health and fitness.

Stretches for Effective Running

The purpose of stretching is to promote recovery. Stretching should be gentle, just until you feel the initial sensation of tension. Never push beyond what's comfortable, it can be harmful. Pay close attention to how you feel and expand your boundaries, but stay within your limits.

The following stretches focus on the muscles that play a key role in running: quadriceps, gluteus, and adductors (inner leg). These stretches will counter the compressive forces of running and promote proper alignment.

Kneeling lunge. This stretch helps relax the compressed areas of the hip and lower back to help your legs recover more effectively. The lunge focuses on the quadriceps and iliopsoas muscles, and the lymph nodes at the lower abdomen. Performing this stretch will stimulate recovery and create elasticity of the quad area while elongating the lower back.

1. From standing, place the top of your right foot on the edge of a chair or the floor behind you.
2. Lower your right knee to the ground, using a towel or cushion for padding.
3. Place your hands on your right knee or the floor.
4. Inhale, lifting your chest and extending your spine.
5. When you exhale, move your lower abdomen back. This rotates your hips to create a stretch in the front of your thigh.
6. Rotate your right hip inward.
7. Hold the stretch for five to twelve breaths.
8. Switch legs and repeat.

During this lunge you should feel a strong, but comfortable, stretch in the front of the leg. If you press too hard, you won't receive the full benefits of the stretch.

Pure hip. Often as an athlete develops back-muscle strength, a corresponding tension and immobility can develop in the lower back. This stretch targets several muscle groups and helps relieve lower-back tension.

1. Lie on your back with your right foot on the wall and the

right knee slightly bent (45 degrees).

2. Cross your left ankle over your right thigh, just above the right knee. The ankle stays flexed.

3. Use your left hand to support your left knee.

4. Maintain this position for five to twelve breaths.

5. Repeat with the other leg.

You can stretch different muscles by moving closer or away from the wall, or by moving your foot farther down the wall.

Inner-leg lengthener. The inner-leg muscles are involved in leg flexion and extension. As a major circulation pathway, the inner leg is prone to injury, so stretch this area with care. This stretch is done with the feet on the wall and the knees bent to reduce the risk of strain.

1. Lie on your back with your hips near a wall, bed, or couch.

2. Place the outside edges of your feet on the wall, with knees bent (45 degrees).

3. Support the inside of your knees with your hands.

4. Focus on moving your toes toward the shins and your heels away from your hips.

5. Bring your chin toward the chest and elongate the neck.

6. Hold this position for seven to ten breaths.

This position should feel good. If it's challenging, bring your legs closer together. Implement steps 4, 5, and 6. As you inhale, expand your chest; when you exhale, press your lower abdomen toward the floor to elongate the lower-back muscles.

Calf with belt. This stretch loosens the foot, challenges the ankle, and releases the back of the knee.

1. Lie on your back and place a strap, towel, or belt around the arch or ball of your left foot.
2. Straighten your left leg and extend your left heel up, stretching the calf. The right leg can be bent or on the floor.
3. Hold the strap with both hands, elbows straight.
4. Hold the stretch for five to twelve breaths.
5. Repeat with other leg.

To fine-tune the stretch, move the outside edge of your foot down, and use the strap to pull the toes toward your shin. Keep your knee straight and move your hip away from the ribs. If your leg is tight, lean your heel on a wall, allowing the lower back to extend.

Hamstring/hip with belt. This stretch releases the tension in the side of the leg and hip to help decompress the hip joint.

1. Lie on your back and place a strap, towel, or belt around the arch or ball of your left foot.
2. Hold the strap in your right hand and place your left arm on the floor, perpendicular to your body.
3. Straighten your left leg and extend your left heel up. Keep the right leg on the floor with your knee bent or straight.
4. Exhale, lower your left leg across your body, moving your left hip away from your ribs. Inhale and raise your leg to the starting position. Repeat three to five times.
5. From starting position, lower your left leg across your body

and hold the stretch for five to twelve breaths. The arm holding the strap stays straight.

6. Repeat with other leg.

Move slowly into the stretch, keep your shoulders on the ground, and rotate your hip away from your ribs to deepen the stretch. Be sure to flex your ankle and straighten your knee, and use the strap to pull the toes toward the shin. Take your time to make small adjustments in the leg position.

Standing hamstring. This stretch safely decompresses the knee, rejuvenates deep hip muscles, and coordinates lower-leg alignment to improve your running gait.

1. Place both hands shoulder-width apart on a wall or the back of a chair.
2. Walk your feet under your hips until your legs are perpendicular to your torso.
3. Arch your lower back.
4. Hold this position for five breaths.
5. Inhale, raise your straightened left leg back to where you feel a stretch; roll your left hip toward the ground.
6. Hold this position for five to twelve breaths.
7. Repeat with the other leg.

Adjust your weight on the standing leg and keep your back arched. As you hold the stretch, drop your hip a little more and practice smooth, relaxed breathing. If you're tight, move your hands up the wall to arch your lower back. The key to these

stretches is to focus on your alignment as you stretch to help promote optimal running alignment.

Tips for the Hopelessly Inflexible

Everyone can enjoy the advantages of stretching—even the hope-
lessly inflexible. If stretching is challenging for you, begin by following two simple steps: Bend your knees and go extra easy.
Bending your knees makes forward stretches feel better, stretches
your hips more effectively (your prime area of mobility), and helps
protect your hamstrings from injury. Throughout your stretching,
keep your breath even and smooth.

Standing-forward bend. This stretch releases your midback,
relaxes your hips, and harmonizes your nervous system.

1. From a standing position, take a deep breath in.
2. As you exhale, bend your knees, lift your chest, and bend
   forward from the hips. When your lower abs touch your
   thighs, release your chest over your legs, drop your head
   and relax.
3. Take a few deep breaths, holding this position.
4. Inhale, lift, and arch your chest two to four inches off your
   legs. Exhale, drop the torso, and fold over your legs.
   Repeat three times.
5. Relax over your legs one final time and hold for four breaths.

Twist. This stretch addresses tight hips and abdominal muscles
while balancing the sacroiliac joint. The less you push, the
better—this is a powerful stretch, so simply relaxing into it

provides the greatest benefits. This stretch is not recommended for those who have a disk injury.

1. Lie on your back with knees bent in toward your chest and arms out to the side, perpendicular to your body.
2. As you exhale, drop your knees to one side, hold and inhale. Exhale as you drop your knees to the other side.
3. Alternate from side to side. Repeat six times.
4. Hold and relax on each side for eight breaths. Think about moving your ribs away from your hips.

Calf Care. As most fast runners know, there can be a price for speed: shin splints. There are many theories about shin splints, but all agree that the calf muscle is involved. To keep your calves healthy, practice daily stretching and self-massage. The best time to stretch your calf is first thing in the morning or a few hours after a workout. Include stretches you can use in different positions such as standing, sitting, and lying down — all positions are effective. Don't worry, you can't overstretch your calves.

The Art of Athletic Recovery

Recovery is crucial for optimal health and performance. It balances the immune and hormonal systems, aids digestion, and facilitates the removal of cellular debris. An effective recovery plan is just as important as a proper training plan.

Passive lunge. The passive lunge addresses a number of powerful leg muscles and helps relieve tension from the quads and adductors (inner leg) to promote lymph circulation. It should feel good and shouldn't require extra energy.

1. Step forward with your right foot; the left foot remains behind with the ball or top of the foot on the ground.
2. Lower your left knee, padding it with a towel or cushion. Allow your left hip to drop toward the floor.
3. Place your hands on the ground on the inside of your front foot.
4. Remain in this position for seven to ten breaths. Focus on dropping your left hip toward the ground. Slightly rotate the back leg in or out to find the tight areas of the inner leg.
5. Lean your weight forward as if you're sliding the left knee on the floor, stretching the thigh. For a greater stretch, put your elbows on the floor.
6. Repeat this series on the other side.

Another option is to do this stretch with your front leg on a chair; your back knee will be off the ground.

Open hips on wall. This stretch promotes overall relaxation and recovery, and focuses on the inner legs.

1. Lie on your back, resting your legs on the wall (if done without a wall, hold your shins).
2. Let your heels slide down the wall toward each other until the bottom of your feet touch.
3. Move your knees away from each other, toward the wall.
4. Place the palms of your hands on the inside of your knees.
5. Hold for seven to ten breaths.

If you're tight, start with your hips farther from the wall. You should feel relaxed; if you don't, change your position. This stretch helps promote recovery of the lymph nodes at the upper leg/lower pelvic area. Don't push this stretch, simply spending time in this position will give you the benefits.

More Recovery Exercises

After working with six Ironman world champions, I realized that their preparation is similar. Everything is measured to fit one intention: to peak on a particular day and be the best. Here are some additional ways to help your legs recover and feel sharp for that important day.

Legs on wall, chest open. This stretch offers benefits without any effort. This is not recommended for people with high blood pressure.

1. Lie on your back with a rolled up towel or pillow under your head.
2. The back of your neck is elongated; chin toward chest.
3. Rest your legs on a wall, couch or chair at least a foot higher than your head (more is okay).
4. Your lower back should be flat on the floor.
5. Place a pillow in between your shoulder blades to open your chest and enhance relaxation.

There is always time to put your legs up. Keep them elevated as often as possible.

Seated pure hip. When your hips are tight, it impairs movement and can stiffen your lower back. Lower-back pain can be devastating: Pros have had to pull out of big races because of lower-back and or sciatic problems. This stretch can help improve hip flexibility and improve circulation and recovery of the adrenal gland, which endures additional stress during training.

1. Sit on a chair.
2. Cross your right shin over your left thigh.
3. Lean your head toward the left knee, and drape your arms over your leg.

This stretch is strong and specific. When you feel tension in your hip, wait and let the hip release before moving deeper. The hip should be opened slowly; never force your stretches.

Your power as a runner is dependent on more than just how much and how far you run. Paying attention to body alignment and mechanics; breathing properly; stretching for flexibility; and allowing your body to recover are all necessary for optimal performance. Incorporate these stretches into your training regimen and feel better, run like a pro, and race and train forever.

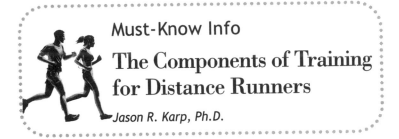

Must-Know Info

The Components of Training for Distance Runners

Jason R. Karp, Ph.D.

One of the things I love most about the sport of distance running is that in the simplicity of putting one foot in front of the other, there is also extreme complexity. When done correctly, it is a scientific endeavor to maximize one's speed and endurance, with many things to address. Here are some of the major components of training.

Mileage

The number of miles you run each week is the most important part of your training. To excel as a distance runner, you need to become as aerobically developed as possible. Running lots of miles serves multiple purposes:

- improves blood vessels' oxygen-carrying capability by increasing the number of red blood cells and hemoglobin
- stimulates the storage of more fuel (glycogen) in the muscles
- increases the use of intramuscular fat to spare glycogen
- creates a greater capillary network for a more rapid diffusion of oxygen into the muscles

- increases mitochondrial density and the number of aerobic enzymes (through the complex activation of gene expression), thereby increasing aerobic metabolic capacity

Research has shown that runners who perform high volumes of endurance training tend to be more economical, which has led to the suggestion among scientists that running high mileage (more than seventy miles per week) improves running economy, the amount of oxygen (VO_2) needed to run at a given speed. Because it's hard to prove cause and effect, it is not entirely clear whether high mileage runners become more economical by running more miles or are innately more economical and can therefore handle higher mileage without getting injured.

The less oxygen you need to run at a specific speed, the better. For example, if Runner A uses forty milliliters of oxygen and Runner B uses fifty milliliters of oxygen while running an eight-minute mile pace, the pace feels easier for Runner A , who is more economical. Therefore, Runner A can run at a faster pace before using the same amount of oxygen and feeling the same amount of fatigue as Runner B.

It is possible that high mileage improves economy due to more repetition of the running movements, which may optimize your biomechanics and muscle fiber recruitment patterns. Additionally, high mileage often leads to weight loss, which would cause a lower oxygen cost to run at a given pace.

Since the duration of effort is one of the key factors that arouse the biological signal to elicit adaptations that will ultimately lead to improvements in your running performance, the amount of time (or number of miles) spent running is more important than the pace at which you run. Therefore, your runs should be easy enough to allow you to increase your weekly mileage over time.

Long Runs

Long runs present a threat to the muscles' survival by depleting their store of glycogen. The human body responds rather elegantly to situations that threaten or deplete its supply of fuel, synthesizing and storing more than what was previously present, thus increasing endurance for future efforts. Empty a full glass, and you get a refilled larger glass in its place (much like at some cocktail parties). The more glycogen you have packed into your muscles, the greater your endurance.

While you should try to not let your long run comprise more than about 30 percent of your weekly mileage, this rule can be broken in the name of necessity if you plan on running only a few times per week. Run at a comfortable, conversational pace (about two minutes per mile slower than 5K race pace, or about 70 to 75 percent of maximum heart rate). Lengthen your long run by one mile each week for three or four weeks before backing off for a recovery week. If you run more than about forty miles per week, or if you run faster than about an eight-minute mile pace, you can add two miles at a time to your long run. Since your legs have no concept of distance—only of intensity and duration—the amount of time you spend on your feet is more important than the number of miles you cover.

Intervals

In the 1960s, famous Swedish physiologist Per-Olaf Åstrand discovered that by breaking a set amount of work up into smaller segments or intervals, you can perform the whole set of work at a higher intensity. Interval workouts alternate high-intensity work periods with low-intensity recovery periods. There are four variables that can be manipulated within an interval workout: time (or distance) of each work period, intensity of each work period, time of each recovery period, and number of repetitions.

Intervals lasting three to five minutes target improvements in your cardiovascular system—specifically, the ability of your heart to pump blood and oxygen to the active muscles. The ability to supply energy for activities lasting more than a couple of minutes depends on the consumption and use of oxygen. Since all distance-running races take longer than two minutes, the consumption and use of oxygen is the energetic basis of endurance performance.

The cardiovascular adaptations associated with interval training increase your VO_2 max, the maximum volume of oxygen your muscles consume per minute. Your VO_2 max represents your aerobic ceiling. You need a high VO_2 max to attain elite-level performances. Think of VO_2 max as your VIP card—a high VO_2 max gains you access into the club. VO_2 max is considered to be the best single indicator of a person's aerobic fitness. It was first measured in humans in the 1920s and has since become the most often measured physiological variable in the field of exercise physiology.

The best way to increase VO_2 max is to run at the speed at which VO_2 max occurs, which is about two-mile race pace for highly trained runners and about 1.5-mile race pace for recreational runners. If using heart rate as a guide, you should come close to reaching your maximum heart rate by the end of each work period.

Intervals lasting from thirty seconds to two minutes target improvements in your anaerobic capacity—the ability to regenerate energy through metabolic pathways that do not use oxygen. These shorter, faster intervals improve your ability to buffer the muscle acidosis that occurs when there is a large dependence on oxygen-independent (anaerobic) metabolism. Since every race distance from 800 meters to 10K has a significant anaerobic contribution, shorter intervals are also an important training component.

Sample Interval Workouts:
- 5 x 800 meters @ VO_2 max pace with 1-to-1 work-to-rest ratio
- 4 x 1,000 meters @ VO_2 max pace with 1-to-1 work-to-rest ratio
- 8 x 400 meters @ mile race pace with 1-to-2 work-to-rest ratio
- 5 x 600 meters @ mile race pace with 1-to-2 work-to-rest ratio

Tempo Runs

Tempo runs target improvements in your lactate threshold (LT), which demarcates the transition between running that generates energy almost purely aerobically and running that includes energy generated from both aerobic and oxygen-independent (anaerobic) metabolism. Thus, the LT represents the fastest speed attainable without a significant anaerobic contribution. Think of the LT as the fastest speed you can sustain aerobically. While VO_2 max has received most of the attention among runners and coaches, the LT is actually more important, as it exerts a greater influence on performance and is more responsive to training than is VO_2 max. While a high VO_2 max is your VIP card, having that VIP card is not enough. To be a great distance runner, you need to have other tools in your physiological arsenal to succeed among the other VIP members. I have tested many athletes in the laboratory with an elite-level VO_2 max, but few of them were capable of running at the elite or even subelite level because they did not have a high LT. Indeed, research has shown that the LT is the best physiological predictor of distance running performance.

The longer the race for which you're training, the more important it is to train your LT so for the marathon and half marathon, the LT should be the focus of your training. The keys to success for the longer distance races are (1) getting your LT pace as fast as you can and (2) being able to run as close to your LT pace as possible for as long as possible. Training the LT shifts it to a faster speed, enabling you to run faster before oxygen-independent metabolism (and fatigue) begins to play a significant role.

I typically use four types of LT workouts with my athletes: (1) continuous runs (2–5 miles) at LT pace; (2) intervals run at LT pace with short rest periods, such as 4 to 6 x 1 mile at LT pace with one minute rest; (3) shorter intervals run at slightly faster than LT pace with very short rest periods, such as two sets of 4 x 1,000 meters at five to ten seconds per mile faster than LT pace with forty-five seconds' rest and two minutes' rest between sets; and (4) medium-long runs (12–16 miles) with a portion at LT pace (for marathoners), such as 4 miles at LT pace + 8 miles easy; 5 miles easy + 3 miles at LT pace + 5 miles easy

+ 3 miles at LT pace; and 10 miles easy + 4 miles at LT pace.

LT pace is about ten to fifteen seconds per mile slower than 5K race pace (or very close to 10K race pace) for runners slower than about forty minutes for 10K (about 80 to 85 percent maximum heart rate). For highly trained and elite runners, the pace is about twenty-five to thirty seconds per mile slower than 5K race pace (or about fifteen to twenty seconds per mile slower than 10K race pace, or about 90 percent maximum heart rate). Subjectively, these runs should feel comfortably difficult.

Weight Training and Plyometrics

Weight training is not as important as the above components for distance runners, but it may still help you improve your performance. An important factor in distance running is to produce and apply muscle force as quickly as possible. A key factor in becoming a better runner is to enhance the steps involved in muscle fiber recruitment and contraction, improving the speed at which muscles produce force. Research has shown that power training, either with heavy weights (e.g., three to four sets of five to six reps using greater than 85 percent of one-rep max) or plyometric exercises—jumping and bounding exercises involving repeated rapid eccentric (lengthening) and concentric (shortening) muscle contractions—improves muscle force production and even improves running economy.

So if you want to become a better runner, integrate these training components into your program. Not only will you be rewarded with higher levels of fitness and new personal records, but you'll also make a complex sport a little simpler.

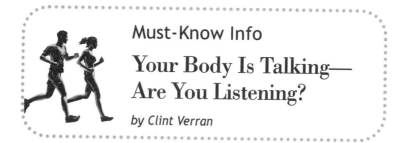

Your Body Is Talking— Are You Listening?

by Clint Verran

One of the greatest aspects of our sport is the concept of the battle against one's self. It doesn't matter how you place if you run faster than you ever have before . . . a personal best (PB)!!! This is why we push ourselves. We push to become better, faster than we were before. Runners are always trying to improve. It's the nature of the sport. Early on, the gains come fast and easy. PBs come almost naturally as our bodies adapt to training stresses. At some point, unfortunately, almost every runner encounters the ultimate PB-killer: running injuries.

Almost any running-based mistake can be overcome. You can start off too fast and recover and still finish a race. You can eat too much before a run and tough it out or make a quick bathroom stop. You can overdress and shed a layer. Once injured, however, the damage is already done. There are no good solutions for running injuries once they occur. Even in the best-case scenario, the runner will need to back down from training so the body can heal. Most often, goals need to be restructured, training becomes severely interrupted, if not halted, and frustration sets in.

Include a Recovery Plan

Nearly every running injury can be traced back to the original training mistake: too much too soon. Runners are naturally wired to push their limits. Newer runners know even less about where or what those limits are. By definition, running injuries are overuse or repetitive-strain injuries. In other words, we runners *work* for our injuries! The act of running is stressful on our bodies. Fortunately, our bodies are usually very good at responding to this stress in a positive and constructive way. Every time we go for a run, we are stressing our muscles, bones, tendons, ligaments, and connective tissues. With an appropriate amount of stress and subsequent recovery, our bodies come back stronger and more resilient for the next stress to be applied. Running injuries occur when the stress outweighs the recovery:

$$STRESS > RECOVERY = INJURY$$

A common mistake that runners make is not planning for recovery. We call our running schedules *training plans*, not *recovery plans*. We seem to think recovery is something that somebody else should do, not us. The reality is that the act of training or *stress* actually makes us worse temporarily. It is during recovery that we improve as runners. Ask yourself this question: Would you rather be 10 percent overtrained and somewhat injured, or 10 percent over-recovered and injury free? The answer should be easy. The key to race-day success is making it to the starting line injury free. To achieve this end, every training plan should incorporate adequate periods of recovery following every period of training.

The difficult part is determining what exactly your recovery should look like. For a beginner, recovery may be a complete day off from exercise. An Olympic-level marathoner may be able to recover with a twenty-mile run. Most of us will fall somewhere in between. Experienced runners should know what it takes for them to recover properly. An example would be a seven-day plan that includes one day completely off from running, as well as two days of easy running following every day of harder running.

Beginners will struggle to learn what their bodies require. Many variables, including age, weight, biomechanics, and even genetics will influence what recovery looks like. The best thing a beginner can do is to seek out the help of a running coach or a veteran runner to help map out a training plan that doubles as a recovery plan.

When to Ignore Pain and When to Pay Attention

Most running injuries are insidious. We don't see them coming because we have learned to ignore our bodies. We expect to have little aches and pains that pop up after beginning a running program. We train ourselves to look past and ignore these nuisances because 99 percent of them go away on their own with zero treatment or training interruption. It's the 1 percent that doesn't go away, ends up getting worse, and interferes with our training that become a problem. Even the experienced runner often has difficulty in determining the difference between the aches and pains that amount to nothing and the few that will bring her running to a screeching halt. Try asking yourself the following questions:

1. Is this pain causing me to alter my natural stride or running form?
2. Does this pain persist beyond running and affect my normal day-to-day activities?
3. Is this pain getting progressively worse?
4. Has this pain stuck around for a week or longer?

If the answer to one or more of these questions is *yes*, you need to wake up and listen to your body! As with other things that affect our bodies, the key to cure is early detection. Here is a quick and easy plan to make most potentially goal-crushing injuries disappear before they have a chance to take you down:

1. If an injury is bad enough to warrant taking a day off (a *yes* answer to one or more of the above questions) . . . proceed to take *two* days completely off.
2. Begin an *icing* program immediately. Apply a bag of ice, cold gel pack, bag of frozen veggies, or stick the injured body part in ice water for fifteen minutes twice a day.
3. Resume your running program once the affected area is free from pain during normal daily activities. If it hurts to walk, you should not be running.
4. For at least one week, run at 50 percent of your normal distance or volume. Avoid intense runs, workouts, or races.
5. Do not try to make up for lost time. A good training plan incorporates enough training stress or redundancy to absorb a week of easy running without completely sacrificing your goals.

6. If after two days of complete rest you continue to have pain, start searching for a mode of cross-training you can do without pain.

It's Back!!!

So, your pain went away and you're back on track with your running program. A week later you are out on a run, and out of nowhere, Mr. Running Injury is back. Now we have a problem. The added rest and recovery, as well as all the icing has not done the trick. Consider now these possible causes of the reoccurring running injury:

Improper footwear. Running in the wrong shoes will eventually injure you. Many foot, ankle, shin, knee, and hip injuries are caused from excessive foot motion. If your foot moves too much or *overpronates*, it will eventually injure you. Contrary to popular belief, no amount of foot, leg, or hip exercises will correct an overpronated foot. If you have a flat foot, you have an overpronated foot. If you don't have a flat foot, you still may overpronate when you run. Overpronation has been linked to plantar fasciitis, ankle pain, Achilles tendinitis, shin pain, stress fractures, knee pain, iliotibial band syndrome, hip pain, bursitis, and low-back pain, just to name a few. If you are not 100 percent confident that you are in the correct shoe, proceed directly to a reputable running specialty store to have your feet evaluated. This single step can be the most important thing you do to enjoy a long, injury-free running career.

Running surfaces. Most running injuries are impact related. We hit the ground with our bodies thousands and thousands of times. Not all ground is the same. Concrete ground is very hard and unforgiving. Many races are run on concrete, and most sidewalks are concrete. Concrete is very abundant, and therefore, convenient for running. But too much concrete running for too long a time will eventually injure you.

Solution: pick the softest, smoothest surface you can find.

Choose asphalt running surfaces over concrete. Choose firmly packed dirt trails over asphalt. The wisdom is self-explanatory. If we can limit the stress of impact from a hard surface, we can train more with fewer injuries. The only instance where training on a harder surface like concrete is advisable is when you are training for an upcoming race or run that will take place on concrete. In this case, make a point of doing at least one run a week on the same surface you will be racing on. I have seen cases where a runner ran 100 percent of the time on a soft squishy treadmill, only to become injured from one hard effort on concrete. It is important to try to simulate your race environment in training from time to time, and running surface is an important part of that training.

What about treadmills? Nothing seems to stir up more controversy among runners than treadmills; many die-hard runners cringe at the thought of running on one. But the fact is, the world is a better place because of treadmills. They are usually the softest, safest running surface a runner has available. Plus, there are many places in the world where running outside can become nearly impossible or unsafe because of weather conditions. They are also great for rehabbing impact-related running injuries.

True, running on a treadmill is not the same as running outside. Your body is not adapting to the forces of impact in the way it has to while running outdoors. It is undeniably boring compared to a beautiful outdoor run. However, when it is a runner's only safe option, a treadmill run beats not running every time. After all, who do you think loves running more: someone who climbs on a treadmill for an hour, enduring boredom and ridicule, or the die-hard who rejects the treadmill and puts on ten pounds waiting for the snow to melt?

Becoming a better runner requires more than just pushing your limits by urging your body to move faster and harder each time you run. In fact, that's a sure recipe for injury. Continually beating your personal best requires listening to your body, properly interpreting the messages of pain, and allowing adequate time for recovery. Your body will thank you with enhanced endurance and superior speed.

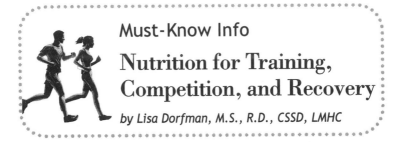

Must-Know Info
Nutrition for Training, Competition, and Recovery
by Lisa Dorfman, M.S., R.D., CSSD, LMHC

W hile successful running is a combination of favorable genes and proper training, the right food can give you the right amount of energy at just the right time. As a competitive distance runner and triathlete for more than two decades, I have seen the impact of food on training, competition, and overall health. I have guided thousands of recreational to Olympic-level athletes to achieve their personal best for more than twenty-five years working as the director of sports nutrition and performance at the University of Miami.

Energy
To be a great runner, your body must be continuously supplied with food energy, called calories. If calorie intake exceeds needs, you'll feel heavy, run slower, and double your risk for injury. If calorie demands increase above and beyond what you consume, you won't be able to maintain speed or distance and recovery will be slow and incomplete. Consult one of the many available sports nutrition books or online guides if you'd like to calculate your own daily energy needs.

Fueling Your Runs

Meeting daily calorie needs for most runners, whether recreational or elite, presents challenges. To succeed as a runner, you need to power your body with healthy, high-energy choices for top performance.

Food Fuel. Carbohydrates, fats, and to a lesser extent, protein are all sources of fuel for running. Your running intensity and duration, fitness level, gender, and diet all impact which fuels you use. Without a diet high in carbohydrates (especially for high-intensity workouts, races, track workouts, or other sprinting), you run on empty. Complex carbohydrates such as whole grain, fruits, and vegetables are more desirable than simple sugars from candies, desserts, and soft drinks because they are higher in vitamins, minerals, fiber, and compounds called phytonutrients that help your body to use fuel, stay fit, recover faster, and reduce the risk for chronic diseases, which, yes, even runners are susceptible to.

Moderate to low-intensity running such as marathoning, ultramarathoning, and slow jogging is fueled primarily by a greater proportion of fat. Fuel from fat should comprise no more than 30 percent of total calorie needs and should come from healthy unsaturated foods, such as peanuts, olives, and their monounsaturated oils; soy foods; nuts like almonds and pistachios; omega 3-rich flaxseed oil and fatty fish like salmon; and trans fat–free unprocessed baked goods and prepared meals.

Protein is important for runners because it helps to build and repair muscle, helps the muscles contract and relax, builds ligaments and tendons that hold muscles and supports bone, and assists with recovery by preventing muscle breakdown. Without adequate dietary protein, you fall apart through injury and illness.

While protein is not your primary fuel for the actual run, it is part of the support system.. Protein from chicken, fish, turkey, red meat, eggs, cheese, milk, and even the only plant source, soy, provides all the essential amino acids—the building blocks of protein that must be supplied by the diet.

How much is enough? Runners following a moderate training program—intensity between 50–70 percent maximum heart rate ([220–age] x .50–.70)—can typically meet their nutrient needs by consuming the following for training:

- 45–55 percent carbohydrates (3 to 5 grams/kg/day)
- 10–15 percent protein (0.8 to 1.0 grams/kg/day)
- 25–35 percent fat (0.5 to 1.5 grams/kg/day)

Kilogram body weight = weight in pounds divided by 2.2. For example, if you weigh 150 pounds then you divide by 2.2 and you get 68 kilograms.

If you're training for a marathon or ultra, or maintain a high volume of running several days a week, then you will need greater amounts of carbohydrates and protein to meet daily needs. A minimum of at least 50 percent, but ideally 60 to 70 percent of total calories from carbohydrates (5 to 8 grams/kg/day), protein (1.2 to 1.7 grams/kg body weight), and fat (20 percent to 30 percent of total calories).

While these percentages are a great starting place for good running nutrition, here are a few tips to keep in mind:

1. Calories should come from a wide variety of foods, representing at least five colors on your plate from all food groups on a daily basis.

2. Eat at least three meals and three snacks throughout the day to sustain energy levels, manage blood sugars, and assist with preworkout and recovery fuel.

3. Choose foods that are as wholesome and fresh as possible with limited additives, colorings, flavorings, and/or processing; with adequate fiber, vitamins, and minerals.

Carbohydrate Fuel

The first source of sugar energy for muscles is from glycogen. When this is depleted, the liver generates glycogen sugars for energy. During long runs that exceed ninety minutes, muscle glycogen drops. When it drops to critically low levels, running at any speed can no longer be maintained. That's when veteran runners can tell you, they've hit the wall—they are exhausted and have immediately stopped running or have drastically reduced their pace. To avoid hitting the wall, it's imperative to eat enough total daily carbs and fuel with carbs before, during, and after running. Here's how:

Prerun fuel. Prerun fuel has been shown to improve performance. The prerun snack helps to maintain optimal levels of blood sugar for muscles and can help restore suboptimal liver glycogen stores that may be called on during long training runs and high-intensity competition. If you train first thing in the morning and cannot imagine consuming anything that early, then make sure your last meal or snack the night before is a good carbohydrate source, such as grains, pasta, rice, potatoes, beans, soy, fruits, and/or vegetables.

The prerun meal formula is 1–4 grams of carbohydrates per kilogram of body weight, eaten one to four hours prior to racing. Prerun foods should be high in carbohydrate, low in fiber, and nongreasy to avoid gut ache. Running on too much food that's high in fat, seasoning, or fiber can cause indigestion, nausea, and sometimes vomiting. Plain spaghetti, toast, cereal, pretzels, bagel, English muffin, PowerBar Performance, SOYJOY, or plain breakfast bars are all examples of easy-to-digest, high-carbohydrate choices. Liquid formulas and high-carbohydrate endurance fuels, such as PowerBar Endurance, Accelerade, and Cytomax, are also acceptable, especially if eating is inconceivable, and they provide an easily digested high-carbohydrate fluid that leaves the stomach faster.

Use what works best by experimenting with foods and beverages during training. Plan ahead by packing favorite powdered drinks, bars, and easy-to-make meals, because you cannot always predict what will be available when you arrive. When I traveled with the U.S. Olympic and Paralympic sailing teams as the sports nutritionist during their competition in China, we packed instant oatmeal, soups, canned tuna, chicken, cereals, rice, as well as bars, gels, etc., because we knew eating would be a challenge. We took home a few gold and silver medals as a measure of our good food prep and eating efforts.

Running fuel. Eating carbohydrates during runs that last longer than one hour also improves performance, speeds recovery, and may help to prevent postrace sniffles. Although this will not prevent fatigue, this will delay it. Eating during exercise has also been shown to spare muscle protein and carbohydrates. Some athletes prefer to use a sports drink, whereas others prefer to eat a solid or gel and consume water.

During a run consume 25–30 grams of carbs every thirty minutes. Many sport drinks, sport gels, gummies, and beans also have about this amount. Exceeding 60–70 grams an hour can cause major gut distress, so keep track of your total sport fuel consumption or you will be searching for more Porta-Johns than you anticipated.

Postrun fuel. On average, only 5 percent of the muscle glycogen used during exercise is resynthesized each hour following exercise. That means at least twenty hours will be required for complete recovery after an exhausting run, provided you get 1.5 to 2 g/kg carbohydrates within thirty minutes after running. The key to great recovery is to consume about 100 grams of carbohydrate within thirty minutes after exercise to maximize muscle glycogen synthesis. Consuming sweeter carbohydrates has been shown to result in higher muscle glycogen twenty-four hours after running compared with the same amount of complex carbohydrates, so sport drinks, bars and shakes, even chocolate milk are ideal postrun recovery choices. Adding about 5 to 9 grams of protein with every 100 grams of carbohydrate eaten after exercise may also increase glycogen resynthesis.

Many runners find it easier and simpler to drink their carbohydrates rather than eat them, or to consume easy-to-eat, carbohydrate-rich foods, such as fruit pops, or fruit slices, including oranges or bananas. Combining protein and carbohydrate in a sport fluid or snack may help to improve performance, increase muscle protein synthesis and net balance, and hasten recovery. A small amount of amino acids, ingested in small amounts alone or in conjunction with carbohydrate after exercise, may stimulate protein synthesis and improve net protein balance at rest, during exercise, and postexercise recovery. This is especially true for older runners. I include CytoSport RTD protein drink or Isopure drink (about one-third of the bottle) to top off each of my water bottles; however you can also use a powdered protein, especially if storage is limited and traveling restrictions apply.

Meeting calorie needs may require the addition of sport bars, drinks, and convenience foods and snacks in addition to whole foods and meals. The best shakes and bars are wholesome, low in fat, rich in protein, and high in fiber for training; higher in carbohydrates, lower in fiber and protein, and lactose free for competition. My bar recommendations are: 100 to 150 calories for those on a 1,200- to 1,800-calorie plan; 150 to 250 calories for those on an 1,800- to 2,400-calorie programs and 250 or more calories for meal replacement or weight gain. Look for a range of 5 to 15 grams of protein, less than 12 grams of sugar for training (up to 30 grams or more for racing), and less than 10 grams of fat. Here are some examples of suitable shakes and bars. There are hundreds to choose from.

Shake and Bar Options	Calories	Protein (g)	Fat (g)	Carbs (g)	Sugar (g)	Fiber (g)
AdvantEdge Shakes	110	17	3	4	3	2
Muscle Milk Light Shake	160	20	4.5	10	0	5
Muscle Milk Light Bar	170	15	6	18	9	4
PowerBar Pria Bar	110	5	3.5	15	9	1
PB & Whey*	140	10	5	14	10	2
SOYJOY Bar*	140	4	6	16	11	3
Vega Vegan Gluten Free, Dairy Free Energy Bar	240	10	10	30	22	6
Vega Vegan Gluten Free, Dairy Free Shake— natural flavor	110	13	3	8	0	7
Accelerade	120	5	1	21	20	0
Clif Bar	240	10	5	44	22	5
Myoplex Lite Bar	190	15	6	25	10	5
PowerBar Endurance	70	0	0	17	10	0
PowerBar Performance	230	8	3.5	45	25	2

*   good for both training and racing

Fluids

Running makes you hot and sweaty, and when heat is generated, it's transferred to the skin in sweat to help cool us off. The daily fluid recommendations for normal healthy individuals are 3.7 liters/day in males (that's 130 ounces, or about 16 cups/day) and 2.7 liters/day for females (95 ounces, or about 12 cups/day). If you work, train, and compete in warm environments, daily fluid needs can increase to more than 10 liters per day. Plain water is not the best beverage to consume because the replacement of electrolytes—like sodium, potassium, calcium, and magnesium—are also essential for complete rehydration.

Prior to running, consume at least 12 to 20 ounces of fluid, two hours before and up until training or competition start. During the run, drink about 4 to 6 ounces every fifteen minutes or 1.5 to 3 miles. Get at least 16 ounces of fluid for every pound lost, and consume about 1.5 times that loss to get adequately rehydrated and prepared for the subsequent run or workout.

Approximately 20 percent of daily fluids can come from foods—fruits and vegetables—while the remaining 80 percent should be from beverages like water, juice, coffee, tea, soup, sports drinks, and soft drinks. Cold water is preferable to warm water because it increases peripheral blood flow, decreases sweat rate, and speeds up gastric emptying time. Alcohol is not an ideal rehydration fluid because it can reduce sugar production from the liver, which can lead to low blood-sugar levels (hypoglycemia) and early fatigue during endurance runs. Alcohol is also not ideal after exercise because of its diuretic effect and adverse effects on blood glucose and glycogen levels. If you must have that postrace beer, be sure to drink equal parts or more of water and/or sports drink to prevent inadequate fluid replacement.

Caffeine actually may help endurance performance, because it mentally reduces fatigue, enhances fat use, and spares muscle glycogen. You can get a kick with just a cup or about 1.5 to 3.0 mg (3.3 to 6.6 mg/kg) of caffeine per pound. If you weigh 150 pounds,

just a 10-ounce cup of coffee can do the trick, so no need for the
double espressos before your next race.

Do You Need More?

Of course, runners need to consume fluids with electrolytes and
shakes and bars with extra carbs, protein, iron, calcium, and other
vitamins and minerals if they don't get it through their diet. But
do you need additional amounts to support the cause? The consensus is that unless you're deficient in a vitamin or mineral, taking supplements will not have a major impact on running
performance. Of course, because of our training and work schedules and the increased energy needs of intense and/or endurance
training, it is nearly impossible to get all forty nutrients, including vitamins and minerals, on a daily basis. If you're a vegetarian,
lactose- or gluten-intolerant, it only makes it more challenging to
meet the essentials.

A diet containing less than one-third of the recommended
daily allowance (RDA) for several of the B vitamins (B1, B2, and
B6) and vitamin C, even when other vitamins are supplemented
in the diet, may lead to a significant decrease in your ability to put
out your highest effort (called VO_2 max) and the anaerobic
threshold in less than four weeks. Hard-training runners may also
run the risk of deficiency in B1, B2, and B6 because these vitamins are involved in energy production. Iron, calcium, magnesium, and potassium are also minerals typically found in low
quantities in the diets of many athletes I see.

The best thing to do is to have your diet evaluated by a sports
dietitian, a registered dietician (RD) that's a certified specialist

in sports dietetics (CSSD). You can find an RD/CSSD in your area at www.scandpg.org. If you decide to look for a supplement on your own, play it safe. Go online to a free dietary analysis website, take a three to seven-day dietary intake and analyze it. If the numbers come up low and you need to supplement, do so with food first. Many of the sport bars, shakes, and drinks are fortified in numerous vitamins and minerals, and you need to eat anyway, so they're a great place to start.

Next, more is not always better. When limited to 100 percent of the RDAs, vitamin supplementation is generally regarded as safe; however, excess amounts of several vitamins may contribute to serious health problems. Check the tolerable upper limits (UL), which have been established for many vitamins at the National Academy of Sciences website. The established dietary reference intakes (DRIs) for vitamins and minerals are listed as a guide for determining nutritional needs at www.iom.edu. Compare those numbers to your supplement to see if the numbers match. If not, save your money and work on the diet, because in the end, the best eaters will make the best runners.

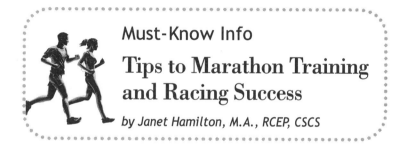

Tips to Marathon Training and Racing Success

by Janet Hamilton, M.A., RCEP, CSCS

There's no one "key" to success when you're talking about training to perform the extraordinary task of running a marathon. Each of us is genetically unique and the individual strengths and weaknesses that make us such an interesting bunch also make it difficult to find a "perfect" cookie-cutter approach to training. When an athlete contacts me for coaching guidance, there are a variety of elements that must be considered. The conversation with a first-timer usually goes something like this:

__Athlete__: I'm interested in training for the _____ marathon. It will be my first marathon.

__Me__: Great, tell me a little more about your recent training history. How long have you been running? How much are you running now and when is this marathon? What is your life schedule like? Have you ever been injured? Do you have any experience with racing at other distances?

What It Really Takes

All too often, the first-time marathoner has no practical understanding of the event. While most runners know that a marathon is a bit over twenty-six miles in length, they have no idea about the necessary preparations for their bodies and are delightfully oblivious to the length of time those preparations will take. Here are a few "rules" for the first-time marathon runner:

Respect the distance you're training for. Depending on your particular race pace, you may be out there running for anywhere from a little over two hours (if you're *really* fast) to six hours or more (if you complete the marathon distance in a run/walk fashion). But, no matter how fast you are—whether you walk it, run it, or crawl it on your hands and knees—twenty-six miles and 385 yards is still twenty-six miles and 385 yards! To accomplish this distance you need adequate endurance, which only comes from putting in some serious training time. An endurance base of forty miles per week with a long run of twenty is pretty much a minimum threshold for successfully completing the marathon, according to most coaches. The consensus among many Road Runners Club of America (RRCA)–certified running coaches is that training for a marathon shouldn't be undertaken until you've been running consistently for several months, preferably a year. Going "from the couch to 26.2" is a risky endeavor.

You should start training for your marathon with a well-established base mileage of about twenty miles per week and a long run of six to eight miles (typical for a fitness runner). Systematically increase your mileage by about 5 to 10 percent per week, and over the course of nine to sixteen weeks of base-building you'll get to a total weekly mileage of about forty miles per week. Picking a marathon date far enough in the future to allow for the inevitable training interruptions due to life, illness, or other constraints is a wise idea. For the runner with a current fitness base of twenty miles per week, an absolute minimum of twenty weeks would allow for a gradual buildup of mileage and a taper period of three weeks before you toe the starting line on race day. Of course, if you start this process with less than twenty miles per week, you'll need substantially longer to build up to race day.

This rule of respecting the distance also plays out for the experienced marathoner. Perhaps you've done one before and your goal is to improve your performance. If you have a particular finish-time goal in mind, you'll improve your odds of success by building your base mileage beyond the minimum, perhaps to sixty miles a week. Running this many miles per week takes time—plenty of time!

> *Athlete: I've been running three days a week. Will that be enough?*
>
> *Me: The more time you can devote to this, the more successful we'll be in getting you to your goal. Can you train more frequently than that?*

Unlike the biology final . . . you can't cram for this test. If you don't do the training, at the very least your results will be less than your potential, and, at the worst, you'll be injured. You're asking your body to make physiological changes on a cellular level and this process is not accomplished overnight—it takes weeks or months to make the physiological changes needed to carry you through the distance. Trying to get by on two or three runs a week is setting the stage for a subpar performance at best. Make the commitment to invest the time needed to do your runs as scheduled.

> *Athlete*: Can I substitute a spin class or boot-camp class for a running day? If so—how many miles can I give myself credit for? What about my elliptical trainer or treadmill, can I use them?
>
> *Me*: The cold hard truth about this is that nothing trains you for running a marathon like running does.

Cross-training is not the same as running. This seems pretty intuitive doesn't it? However, there are many athletes who try to "equate" minutes on a bike or an elliptical trainer or time in the pool to miles of running. There's nothing intrinsically wrong with biking or elliptical machines or swimming. It's just *not* the same as running from a biomechanical or physiological standpoint. You'll get a cardiovascular benefit (your heart and blood vessels will be stronger) but you won't get the same physiological adaptations in your muscles, tendons, bones, or nerves. You can't expect to succeed at your best in a marathon if you don't get out there and run. The corollary to this is that running on the treadmill is *not* the same as running over Mother Earth. Whenever possible, try to do the majority of your running on the same terrain you plan to race on (roads, trails, etc.).

Now that the stage is set and you understand the magnitude of the event you are taking on, it's time to get to the day-to-day planning process. The first-time marathoner, and sometimes even the experienced marathoner, is often surprised by how important it is to manage training paces and loads to minimize injury risk.

Proper pacing is crucial. Train at a pace that's most likely to stimulate the physiological adaptations you need to succeed. It's probably easier than you think. Most runners, left to their own devices, run at paces that are inappropriately fast. They tend to go out the door at or near race pace on every run, and in the process they not only increase the risk of injury but they potentially shortchange the physiological adaptations they're trying to achieve. They teach their bodies to burn fuel rapidly, rather than teaching them to become more *efficient* at burning fuel. When you exercise at a high intensity, you have to utilize fuel at a higher rate. The fuel best suited for this is carbohydrate (in the form of glycogen) and the process produces by-products (lactate is one) at a high rate. Lactate can be recycled and used as a source of fuel *if* you are exercising at a rate that allows your body to utilize the lactate as fast as it's being produced. If you're producing it faster than it can be used, it is sent out into your bloodstream to be shuttled to other areas of your body. A high level of circulating blood lactate is associated with a limited time to exhaustion. The trick here is to make more of the little cellular organs that like to use lactate for fuel—the mitochondria. By training at paces that allow your body to use lactate for fuel (read that as "easy, aerobic paces"), you'll stimulate your body to make more mitochondria and get better at utilizing the lactate and other by-products that are being produced. When training at easy aerobic paces, you become a much more efficient engine and you utilize a slightly greater proportion of fat for your fuel source.

So, what is an easy pace? A good rule of thumb is to run at a pace that's about 80 percent of what you could race *that distance* at. So your "easy pace" for a six-mile run might be 80 percent of your 10K race pace, and for a sixteen-mile run it might be closer to 80 percent of your half marathon pace! By easing your pace on training runs you may find your body becoming more efficient and therefore find yourself racing better! Relax, enjoy the journey—remember, they don't hand out prizes for the best training run.

In addition to the pacing element, athletes often are surprised to know that varying their training distance from day to day will also enhance their performance. The reason is simple; *recovery is part of training*. If you alternate a relatively longer run one day with a shorter run the next, you'll be allowing time on that short day for some active "recovery." It's during the recovery that the physiological adaptations can take place. Overload (longer) days stimulate the change; recovery (shorter) days provide the opportunity for it to take place.

Staying Healthy and Injury-Free
Somewhere along the line in training, the conversation with our first-time marathoner turns to running-related injury.

> ***Athlete***: *Lately I've been feeling my _____. It's not bad—I can run through it . . . but I just wondered what stretches I should be doing to make this go away.*
>
> ***Me***: *Unfortunately, you can't stretch away an injury. We have to get to the root of the problem and you may need to take a few days off to give the tissue some time to heal. How long have you been feeling this?*

Athlete: Only a day or two—and the symptoms are really minor.

Perhaps the most crucial guideline for injury avoidance (and all too often overlooked by the zealous runner) is to tune in to any symptoms you may notice, no matter how small they may seem. If you catch injuries early—when they're just a "whisper" of a symptom—you'll be able to intervene quickly and potentially keep that whisper from becoming a shout. This is a difficult lesson to learn, but best learned early in your career as a runner. Runners are generally reluctant to take time off training, especially with a key event looming on the horizon, but the sooner you act, the shorter the time off will be. Along those lines, the wise runner will avoid masking their symptoms by taking medications that are analgesic in nature. This includes over-the-counter anti-inflammatory medications which all have a strong analgesic (painkiller) component. Most of the injuries sustained by runners are now thought to be degenerative rather than inflammatory in nature, so not only do you inhibit your ability to feel (and therefore heed) your symptoms, you're also using a drug that doesn't help the underlying injury because the cause is probably not inflammatory in nature to start with.

Often the best defense against running-related injuries is good strength. Many studies on running-related injuries point to the fact that strong muscles are better able to withstand forces and resist fatigue and offer some protection from injury. A bit of time each week working your lower back and abdominal muscles as well as the sides of your hips can go a long way toward making you more efficient and injury-resistant. You can't "stretch away" an injury, but by maintaining adequate flexibility and strength in all your muscles you may be able to avoid injury—or at least shorten your road to recovery.

As the training progresses and the mileage increases it becomes more and more important to fuel and hydrate your body well on a regular basis. You can't get top performance from a race car if you put low octane fuel in it, and you can't get top performance out of a human body if you don't fuel it well. There aren't any magic supplements or fuels out there (contrary to advertising claims) that will enhance your performance better than eating a healthy and balanced diet full of whole grains, fruits, and vegetables, with lean protein and a little healthy fat added to the mix. Entire books have been written on nutrition for runners and are well worth the time you will invest to read them. Suffice it to say that training for a marathon is not the time to be cutting calories in an effort to lose weight.

Fuel the body so that it has the needed building blocks to make the physiological adaptations you're asking for and the necessary nutrients to fuel your exercise. Stay well hydrated all the time. Plan to take water with you on runs that last longer than about forty-five minutes (especially in hot climates) or be willing to run a route that has water available along the way. When the long run exceeds two hours in length you'll find that taking in some carbohydrate fuel during the run helps delay the onset of fatigue. Commercially available carbohydrate supplements are available at your local running store, or you can use simple snacks like jelly beans. Whatever sits well on your stomach works just fine.

By training consistently and building mileage gradually our first-time marathoner is ready for the distance on race day.

> *Athlete: Tomorrow is my race, and I was thinking that it would be a good strategy to try to run a little faster in the first half when I'm fresh. That way if I slow down in the second half I'll still get my goal time.*
>
> *Me: Quite the contrary. Avoid the common error of going out too fast in the beginning of the race, thinking you're going to give yourself some "padding" in the process.*

Going out a minute a mile too fast in the beginning will very likely cost you two minutes a mile in the later stages. There's a common term among distance athletes: "hitting the wall." That's the feeling you get when you've burned up your available fuel (by going out too fast) and your body simply feels as if you've just run into a brick wall. The best way to avoid the wall is to meter out your fuel supply wisely by running the race with a close eye on your pacing.

Marathons are a wonderful and challenging experience. Train well, stay healthy, and enjoy the journey through training all the way to the finish line!

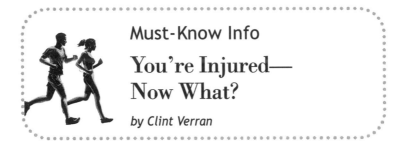

Must-Know Info

You're Injured—
Now What?

by Clint Verran

Y ou followed the training plan to the letter, yet you have a running injury. It happens to the best of us. Welcome to the dark side. You thought your training plan was challenging? Get ready for the ultimate test of a runner's mettle—managing your running injury.

What was once merely an ache or a pain has interrupted or put a halt to your running. The first step to getting through the quagmire of injury is figuring out exactly what is going on with your body. This is harder than it sounds. To properly treat your injury, it is necessary to categorize it. The three most commonly injured structures are muscle, bone, and connective tissue.

What Is Hurting?

Muscle: Muscle tissue is constantly being broken down and built back up. It's when a muscle get pushed too far that problems arise. Commonly injured ones include calves, shin muscles, thigh muscles (hamstrings and quadriceps), and gluteal muscles.

Most muscular injuries heal relatively fast.

Bone: Bone injuries are serious. Most running-related bone injures are stress fractures. When the stresses from running exceed the re-modeling rate, stress fractures occur. Stress fractures can develop slowly over time or they can pop up suddenly. Stress fractures typically masquerade as muscle pain. One of the key characteristics of a stress fracture is a deep-seated dull ache that worsens with weight bearing or impact. The shinbone (tibia) is the most common site for stress fractures with the long bones of the foot (metatarsals) as a close second. Other bones to watch out for include the thigh bone (femur) and the pelvis.

X-rays are rarely useful in diagnosing stress fractures. If you think you might have a stress fracture, ask your doctor for a bone-scan or an MRI. The most common cause of stress fractures is TMTS along with a contributing biomechanical issue such as an overly high-arched foot. Unfortunately, the only effective treatment for a bone injury is nonrunning rest. Initially, most forms of cross-training should be excluded as well. Swimming or pool running is the best choice. After a few weeks, a stationary bicycle will work. Elliptical trainers add even more weight bearing and can be useful once walking and cycling are pain-free. The amount of time before returning to running depends on the size of the bone and the runner's age. Smaller bones in younger people heal faster. For example, a seventeen-year-old may be able to return to running after a metarsal stress fracture in as little as four weeks. A sixty-year-old with a pelvic stress fracture may require twelve months.

Connective Tissue: Tendons, ligaments, fascia, and cartilage make up the connective tissue category and are the most commonly injured tissues. Achilles tendonitis, plantar fasciitis, Iliotibial band syndrome (ITBS), patellar tendonitis, runner's knee, compartment syndrome, bursitis, and many other injuries can be classified as connective tissue injuries. These injuries present challenges on many fronts. They lack direct blood flow, making the healing process inherently slow. It is also impossible to strengthen connective tissue, and in many cases, once damaged, it may never return to its pre-injury state. Early detection becomes very important when dealing with a potentially chronic connective tissue injury. These injuries often have a biomechanical origin. A good example is an overpronated or flat foot. A runner with runner's knee can strengthen his legs all he wants, but if the torsion caused by overpronation is not addressed, all other time spent in therapy may be time wasted.

In real life, most running injuries involve a combination of issues. For example, a common injury for beginner runners is shin splints. The average case of shin splints involves pain along the inside of the shinbone (tibia). This part of the shinbone serves as the origin attachment for a muscle known as tibialis posterior. This muscle acts to help control the foot at impact as well as absorb shock. When a runner increases training, this muscle must worker harder. More foot strikes equals more work for the muscle. Every time the muscle contracts it pulls hard along the inside edge of the shinbone. This pulling action can irritate the connective tissue lining of the bone known as the periosteum. With enough stress, the underlying shinbone itself can fail resulting in a stress fracture. The other end of the muscle attaches to a tendon at the muscle-tendon junction. This junction is a weak link in the system and is a common place for pain or injury. The tendon then attaches to a bone in the foot that can fail after repeated stress. A flat or overpronated foot makes more work for this system. Therefore, a biomechanical imperfection coupled with increased training stress can easily create a perfect storm of injury: first a muscular, then a connective tissue, then finally a bone injury.

Treatment

The biggest mistake we make is not differentiating symptoms from the cause or mechanism of injury. Symptoms usually include pain, swelling, stiffness, soreness, and sometimes, bruising. The cause can include too-much-too-soon, improper footwear, poor running surfaces, biomechanics, or weakness, and usually a combination of two or more of these issues. The key to proper treatment is quickly addressing both the symptoms *and* the cause.

Treating symptoms is the easy part. There is a miracle agent that dramatically decreases swelling, reduces pain, promotes healing, and, best of all, is almost free: ICE! Cold therapy is an essential part of the injury-treatment process, is most crucial in the early stages of treatment, and is the best way to get swelling or inflammation under control. Ice the affected area for fifteen minutes, twice a day. If you are cross-training or able to "run-through" your injury, you must ice immediately following exercise. Continue to ice your injury all the way through the treatment process, and don't stop until you are back to pain-free running.

The most powerful therapy we possess is our body's own healing ability. Yet rest is a four-letter word, especially to runners.

Most runners would rather be shocked by a taser than have to rest. Rest is the most effective form of treatment because it addresses both symptoms and cause, and it absolutely needs to be a major part of your treatment plan. "Relative rest" that substitutes alternative forms of activity for activities that aggravate the symptoms, along with ice may be all that is needed for the body to start repairing itself. In the case of a more serious injury, treatment might include several months of nonrunning.

Most running injuries have an inflammatory component, causing swelling, pain, and stiffness. Therefore, they respond quite quickly to nonsteroidal anti-inflammatory drugs (NSAIDS) like ibuprofen, aspirin, and naproxen. This can be good and bad. Small doses of over-the-counter NSAIDS coupled with rest and ice over a short period of time can be an effective strategy to get a running injury under control. During this time, the runner must seek out the underlying cause and address it. If not, he is destined to suffer the same injury over and over again. All too often, runners will use NSAIDS as a cheap fix for their injury. NSAIDS are inherently unsafe and should never be used as an enabling agent. If you need to take NSAIDS to run, you should not be running.

There is no shortage of self-help injury gizmos in today's market place. As a general rule, most braces, straps, splints, supports, and bands are of little help in actually fixing a running injury. Some over-the-counter arch-supporting inserts can successfully address an overpronated or flat foot. I am also impressed by the foam roller's ability to keep muscle and fascia knots from becoming problematic.

Treating the cause is relatively easy. First you will need to revisit your training plan. Your original plan injured you; now you have the added challenge of trying to get back on track. Depending on how long your injury took to resolve, you may or may not need to adjust your goals, particularly your near-term goals.

Use this injury as a learning experience. You now have a better understanding of how your body works, how it is supposed to feel, and how the warning signs of injury present. If a biomechanical issue contributed to your injury, it must be addressed or you are only destined to relive the injury in the future. Fixes might include a more supportive or more cushioned shoe, foot orthotics to control overpronation, a stretching program for your super-tight IT bands, or a core-strengthening program. If you determined that your injury was impact-related, you may need to alter the surfaces you choose to run on. If running on concrete every day caused your metatarsal stress fracture, you need to find somewhere softer to run.

Running injuries are an ugly side effect of training errors, biomechanical issues, or probably both. Ignoring them will *not* make them go away. Take action to quickly identify the nature, severity, and most important, the cause of the injury. Don't be afraid to get help. A doctor or therapist with extensive experience helping runners can prove invaluable. Be prepared to take an appropriate amount of rest. And don't give up on your running! It is an important part of your life now and certainly can be for years to come.

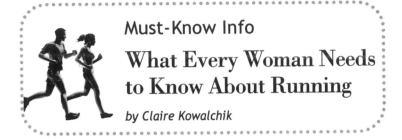
Ten years ago, I was enjoying one of the best jobs imaginable as managing editor of *Runner's World* magazine. I wrote and edited stories on one of my favorite subjects, worked with a terrific staff, always ran with friends during my lunch hour, traveled around the world for running events, met famous runners, even had the opportunity to attend the Olympic Trials. I left that amazing job to write a book about women's running from a small room in my home and for very little money. Why? Because I believe so strongly in the value of running to women's lives, and I wanted to give the gift of running to as many women as possible.

Running is the perfect physical activity for women who do too much—which is most of us. The number one reason women give for not exercising regularly is that they have no time. Running is the most efficient and most accessible way to cardiovascular fitness, and not just because you can get in an intense workout in thirty minutes or less, but because it's so simple. You can do it anywhere, anytime, no skill required. And the only "technical" equipment you need is a good pair of well-fitting running shoes and a sports bra.

And this efficient physical activity offers so many benefits that are particularly important to women. Running protects us from cardiovascular disease—the number one killer of women; prevents osteoporosis better than resistance training, according to a recent study published in the *Journal of Strength and Conditioning Research*; relieves the stress of our busy days; helps to lift depression, which we suffer from in greater numbers than men; improves our body image; builds confidence and self-esteem; may ease the symptoms of menopause; and for those of us who never had the athleticism or encouragement to play sports in school, running offers an opportunity for competition.

Now that your excitement for this sport has been either reinvigorated or newly ignited, let's look at several important ways every woman runner can increase her running success for years to come.

Run smart. Some would tell you that women are more prone to injury than men, and we do have a couple of potential disadvantages. We have wider hips in relation to the rest of our body than men do. This brings greater inward pressure on the knee and outward rotation of the shinbone as we run, making us more vulnerable to knee problems, shin splints, and stress fractures. In addition, our joints tend to be more lax than men's, and those joints become even looser with changes in hormones.

But do women suffer more injuries than men? In 2000, the Centers for Disease Control (CDC) undertook a major review of research to examine injuries in women who exercise. They looked at studies of women in the military who undergo rigorous training (which includes marching and running), as well as studies of the civilian population. In military basic training where men and women follow the same training regimen, incidence of injury was twice as high among women. For stress fractures, in particular, incidence was 210 times that of men. But when the researchers looked at studies of civilian runners, rates of injury were similar among women and men.

Further digging showed that, overall, men who enter the military have greater strength and cardiovascular fitness than women, which explained the lower risk of exercise-related injury. The researchers concluded that among the civilian population, women could design their training to suit their fitness level, hence the parity in injury among women and men. The learning? When we train appropriately for our fitness level, we avoid injury.

What does this mean for you?

Increase mileage gradually. Hold to a particular level of total weekly mileage for about three weeks; then add 10 to 15 percent of that total mileage.

Increase frequency gradually. If you are new to running or returning to running after a break, start with three or four days a week and build from there. And even if you run six or seven days a week, be sure to alternate longer and shorter runs with harder and easier ones to give your body the rest it needs, both to recover from physical exertion and to build fitness.

Step up intensity slowly, too. Run at a pace that allows you to have a conversation. With this as your only guide, your pace will not necessarily be the same every day. On days when your body is stronger, you'll run faster; when you're tired, you'll run slower, and that's as it should be—that's how you avoid injury and how you build fitness.

If you want to get faster, you will need to run faster, but if you run fast every day, you'll burn out or get injured, or both. There are many different ways and training schedules for improving speed; find a plan and follow it, or find a running coach who has a good reputation.

Listen to your body and your mind. When you are running too much or too hard, you'll feel tired, maybe even irritable. Running will be sluggish and feel difficult. Cut back on your mileage or intensity—you may be wearing yourself down rather than building yourself up.

Learn how to interpret pain. Muscle soreness and aches often come with increases in mileage or intensity or even a run over hilly terrain. Pain in your joints, sharp pain, and pain that persists or worsens as you run are signs of the onset of injury. Take a break from running and see a doctor if the pain persists.

Build your strength. Given our tendency toward knee problems and stress fractures—strength training is essential. A strength program for your whole body is best.

Recent research, including a study published in the May/June 2009 issue of *Sports Health*, indicates that weak hip and gluteus muscles (glutes) can lessen the stability of the legs while running, making you more vulnerable to knee injuries and other problems of the lower leg. Include hip stabilization exercises in your strength-training regimen. At www.wonderhowto.com you can find a video by Dave Scott, former world-class triathlete and now coach, showing four exercises for the hips and glutes that will benefit runners. Or, you might try Pilates or a core-strengthening routine that includes exercises for hips and glutes.

Eat to win. Sports nutritionists find that women runners often fall short of the recommended 1,300 milligrams (mg) of calcium a day. Calcium plays an important role in muscle contractions and heartbeat and of course it is essential to bone strength. We absorb calcium better from foods than from supplements. Try to include low-fat dairy products—milk, yogurt, cheese—in your diet every day. But don't consume your day's calcium in one sitting. Your body can only absorb 500 mg at a time.

Nutritionists also find iron deficiency to be more common among women athletes than male athletes. We lose iron through sweat and during menstruation. And some iron gets broken down in our tissue as our feet pound the pavement when we run. These losses when combined with a diet low in iron-rich foods can leave us short on this mineral, which carries oxygen throughout the body for energy production. Signs of iron deficiency include fatigue, irritability, decreased endurance, and you may find that you become chilled easily. If you suspect iron-deficiency anemia, see your doctor.

Meat, poultry, and fish provide the most absorbable form of iron. If you are vegetarian, eating foods high in vitamin C with vegetarian sources of iron will increase absorption. Do not take iron supplements without the advice of a physician as overloading on iron can cause health problems. The recommended daily intake is 18 mg.

Women concerned about their weight often avoid dairy products and red meat and may restrict carbohydrates. But carbs have been and always will be the fuel of athletes. Make sure you consume at least 50 percent of calories from carbohydrates—fruits, vegetables, cereals, as well as breads and pastas.

Concern about weight may cause some women to consume too few calories of any kind. The goal may be thinness or faster race times but some women restrict calories to the point of developing what's called the female athlete triad, where disordered eating causes low energy, amenorrhea, and weak bones, which in turn, may lead to stress fractures and osteoporosis. Strive to maintain a body mass index (BMI) in the acceptable range between 18 and 25 (BMI calculators are easy to find online). Eating to win doesn't just mean eating to fuel your running but also to enhance your health.

Run safe. Maybe you love listening to music while you run. But please save the iPod for the treadmill. Wearing a headset while you run makes you less aware of your surroundings and more vulnerable. The more vulnerable you are, the greater your risk for being attacked. Run with awareness. If you hear someone running behind you, turn around and look to show that you know he's there. Heed your reaction if you get an uneasy feeling about the person, and go somewhere safe—immediately.

One of the best ways to stay safe on your run is to go with a friend, but when you go alone, consider these precautions:

- Let someone know where you are going and how long you expect to be gone.
- Carry identification.
- Avoid running in isolated areas.
- Do not run the same—predictable—route every time.
- Avoid engaging with strangers.
- Run during daylight hours; most assaults occur between 6:00 PM and 6:00 AM.

If someone should attack you, fight back in whatever way you can—kicking, screaming, hitting, biting—and run when you get free. According to experts from Arming Women Against Rape & Endangerment (AWARE), attackers choose women they see as vulnerable and weak and whom they don't expect to fight back. Doing the unexpected throws them off guard and often scares them away. Run in the opposite direction an attacker is running or driving, waving your arms in the air to attract attention, and run into open areas such as parking lots or fields. Do not run into alleys, wooded areas, buildings, or enclosed areas where you can be cornered. If you do get cornered, fight to get away.

Run through PMS, pregnancy, and menopause. Your period hits—you feel bloated, tired, you have cramps. Take two Tylenol and go for a run. Though experts have yet to pinpoint an exact relationship between hormones and exercise that is consistent among all women, many women find that they run their best during the first days of their menstrual cycle, reporting that running can seem surprisingly effortless. It is the week prior to the beginning of the menstrual cycle when women often report feeling that their running feels labored. Every woman's body behaves differently, though, so to understand the effects of your hormonal cycle on your running and training, keep a journal and look for trends.

We do know that during pregnancy your body produces the hormone relaxin, which loosens the pelvic joints and affects the laxity of other joints as well. This may increase risk of injury during pregnancy, but if you are comfortable with the idea of running while pregnant and have your obstetrician's approval, you can continue to run and enjoy its rewards. Note the word "continue." Pregnancy is not the time to begin an intense physical activity like running.

And because running is physically intense, it is important to your health not to do it sporadically but to maintain consistency, running a minimum of three times a week. Many women run throughout their entire pregnancy; others choose to stop after the second trimester when running may become uncomfortable. Listen to your body and do what feels right. Early on you may maintain your prepregnancy mileage and frequency, but eventually you'll want to cut back. Run at a pace that is comfortable and allows conversation.

And besides the normal safety precautions, such as staying well-hydrated and steering clear of slippery or uneven surfaces, be sure to stop if you feel fatigue, pain, or notice any vaginal bleeding; choose a route that offers opportunities for "bathroom breaks"; and run in a neighborhood or populated area where you can easily get assistance if you need it.

Women who run during pregnancy feel healthier and have more energy than those who don't exercise at all—benefits that are likely to continue long after the baby is born. A report in the *American Journal of Obstetrics & Gynecology* found that women who continued a vigorous weight-bearing exercise program like running during pregnancy were much more likely to maintain a high level of physical activity after pregnancy than those who stopped exercising, resulting in better cardiovascular health and fitness as they approached menopause.

Once women have passed through their reproductive years, can running ease the symptoms of menopause? Again, we have only anecdotal evidence to go by. Some women swear that running prevents hot flashes, mood swings, and sleepless nights. What we do know is that running helps us manage our weight, keeps our cardiovascular system strong, prevents osteoporosis, lifts our spirits, gives us energy, and offers many other benefits that enhance health and happiness.

Make running a priority. Researchers at Stanford University wanted to discover the long-term effects of running on health and longevity. So over a twenty-one-year period, they studied a group of 538 people who ran regularly and a group of 423 people who never exercised. All participants were fifty years of age or older. By the nineteenth year of the study, 15 percent of the runners had died, compared with 34 percent of the sedentary group. At the twenty-one-year mark, the runners showed better cardiovascular fitness, increased bone mass, less physical disability, even improved thinking, learning, and memory. Even as the active group gave up running for less strenuous activities like walking as they moved into their seventies and eighties, their good health endured while that of the sedentary group declined.

Yes, we women are busy, busy, busy, but the evidence is clear that we must make time for running. Having a friend to run with is a strong motivator to get out the door. And each of you can make the other accountable to a plan of consistency. Setting a race goal can help you stick to a schedule of training. Maybe all you need is a running log where you can see your accomplishment. Or maybe the motivation is simply remembering the breeze in your hair, the sun on your face, fresh air, and the energy of the run pulsing through your body. A long-time friend and runner once said to me, "I've never gone on a run that I regretted." After every run I make, her words ring true.

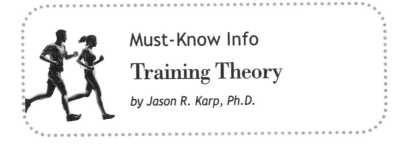

Must-Know Info
Training Theory
by Jason R. Karp, Ph.D.

From an evolutionary perspective, an organism's structural design evolves to cope with the stresses to which it is subjected and is regulated by its functional demand. While our bodies' structural form has developed from millions of years of evolution, structural changes also occur in the short term in response to a training program. For example, with the right stimuli, bones increase their density, muscle fibers increase their metabolic machinery, and cardiac muscle grows larger. If structure and function are matched to the demand, it's logical to assume that if we increase the demand, we'll ultimately increase the amount of change that takes place to keep pace with the increased demand. And that's exactly what happens with runners.

Following a training stress, your body adapts and physiologically overcompensates so that if the same stress is encountered again, it does not cause the same degree of physiological disruption. In short, your body adapts to be able to handle the stress. Following the adaptation, your body can do more work. The aim of training, therefore, is to introduce training stimuli so higher and higher levels of adaptation are achieved. Think of these training stimuli as small threats to the body's survival. If you repeatedly threaten the body's survival, you will make adaptations to assuage the threat. A classic example of this is the long run of marathoners. Repeatedly running for long periods of time (longer than two hours) presents a threat to the muscles' survival by depleting their storage of preferred fuel (glycogen, the stored form of carbohydrates). If you run out of fuel, the muscles say, "Hey, this body is running for so long that I don't have any more fuel. I won't be able to survive. If this activity becomes a regular habit, I need to make more fuel." So, guess what happens? When you consume carbohydrates following your long run, you respond to the empty tank by synthesizing and storing more glycogen than usual in your skeletal muscles, thus increasing your storage of fuel (and therefore your endurance) for future efforts. Pretty elegant.

Unfortunately, our ability to adapt to a training stimulus doesn't keep occurring indefinitely. There will come a point, specific to each runner, when more training does not lead to more adaptations and faster race times. For example, research has shown that mitochondrial density is highly modifiable, and that the number of mitochondria increases in response to endurance training. Mitochondria are structures inside cells that convert nutrients to energy (aerobic metabolism). The more you have, the greater your physical endurance; in other words, the higher your mitochondrial density, the farther and better you can run.

However, there is a threshold above which further increases in training volume do not result in further increases in mitochondrial density. The main difference between Olympic athletes and the rest of us is that Olympic athletes continue to make physiological adaptations up to a very high level of work (more than 100 miles per week). Most of us will stop adapting far short of 100 miles per week.

There is also a load of training, specific to each runner, that leads to injury. The human body is great at adapting to stress *as long as that stress is applied in small doses.* When the stress is too severe, or not enough recovery has preceded the new stress, injury can result. Another unique characteristic of Olympic runners is that they can tolerate very high training loads without getting injured. Most runners would likely suffer injury if they attempted to run 100 miles per week.

How Do We Adapt?

While runners often hear about training and adaptation, how does that adaptation occur? How much you adapt to a training stimulus ultimately depends on how responsive your cells are to signals. Muscle cells are able to detect all kinds of signals—mechanical, metabolic, neural, and hormonal, which are amplified and transmitted via signaling cascades and lead to the events involved in gene expression. This signaling is fast, occurring within minutes of completing a workout. Signaling results in the activation of proteins that bind to a specific part of DNA and control the transfer of genetic information from DNA to RNA.

When you begin a training program, you will experience many signaling responses and subsequent adaptations. However, continual training at the same level decreases the training-specific signaling responses involved in the adaptations to training. In other words, if your training stays the same, you can expect your performances to stay the same. For example, if you run fifteen miles on Sunday morning when you're used to running only twelve, you will send a strong signal to make specific adaptations (increase in mitochondria, muscle glycogen content, etc.). If you continue to run fifteen miles every Sunday for a period of time, you'll continue to send signals to make adaptations until those adaptations are fully realized. After you have run fifteen miles so many times that you have become habituated to it, a fifteen-mile run will no longer be enough of a stimulus to initiate any further adaptations. Therefore, if you want to force more adaptations, you must run longer than fifteen miles (or run the miles faster). To become a faster runner, you have to gradually and systematically increase the amount of stress so that you increase the signaling response.

Specificity of Training

Functional changes take place only in the organs, cells, and intracellular structures that are stressed during physical activity. In other words, if you want bigger biceps, doing squats won't help. Muscles adapt to the specific demands placed on them. In addition to the physiological changes that take place inside your muscles, there is also a motor unit (muscle fiber) recruitment aspect to training. Your brain needs to learn to communicate with your muscles to perform a specific task, and your muscles need to learn to produce force at specific joint angles, which influence the amount of force muscles can produce. Therefore, you need to train the entire movement pattern, rather than the strength or endurance of individual muscles or single joint movements. That's why running won't help you become a better cyclist any more than riding a bike will help you become a better runner. The movement patterns of the two sports are completely different and therefore differ in their motor unit recruitment patterns and their muscles' ability to produce force. For example, cyclists use their hip flexors and quadriceps muscles at short lengths due to their pronounced flexed posture at the hip joint, while runners use their hip flexors and quadriceps muscles at long lengths due to their upright posture. The chronic use of these muscles at different lengths by these athletes results in different relationships between muscle length and the forces they can produce at those lengths.

The same concept holds true for cross-country running compared to track or road running. When training for cross-country races, you should run as much as you can on cross-country courses that include grass and dirt. This includes all of your formal workouts as well, like tempo runs and intervals. You need to accustom your muscles and tendons to cross-country terrain. Good runners will run well regardless of the terrain, but doing all of your workouts on a track to prepare for a cross-country race is like a tennis player practicing on a hard court to prepare for a tournament on a clay or grass court. The way a tennis player's feet move and the way the ball bounces on a clay or grass court are different from on a hard court, just like running on a track is different from running on grass fields and dirt trails, where there is more side-to-side ankle movement. You need to train on the surface you plan to race on.

While training movement certainly needs to be specific to your racing environment, the specificity of training principle does not always hold when it comes to the intensity of running. Although the specificity of training principle would dictate that if you want to get faster for a 5K you should train at a 5K race pace as much as possible, the majority of a distance runner's training is performed at a low intensity, much slower than race pace. Unlike other sports, endurance sports are volume based. And to handle a lot of volume, you have to run slow most of the time. To run fast, you first must spend a lot of time running slow. Running at 5K race pace every day is not the best way to improve your 5K time.

Recovery

Recovery may be the most overlooked aspect of training. Most runners focus on miles and pace. Improvements in fitness, however, occur during the *recovery* period between training sessions, not during the training itself. Positive physiological adaptations occur when there is a correctly timed alternation between stress and recovery. When you finish a long run or interval workout, you are weaker, not stronger. How much weaker depends on the severity of the training stress. If the stress is too great and/or you don't recover before your next workout or race, your performance and your ability to adapt to subsequent training sessions will decline. The faster and more complete your recovery, the more you will get out of your training and racing. While understanding how to cause specific biochemical and physiological changes is the science of training, understanding how to manipulate stress and recovery in an organized and systematic training program to get the greatest adaptation possible is the art of training.

So before you go out the door for your next run, design your program with these concepts in mind. And if you train smart enough, not only will you be rewarded with new personal records, you may even be able to make more adaptations and cheat evolution.

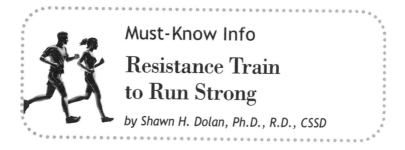

Must-Know Info
Resistance Train
to Run Strong
by Shawn H. Dolan, Ph.D., R.D., CSSD

Resistance training was once thought to be an activity only for those involved in competitive weight lifting, power lifting, or bodybuilding. However, as time has passed, athletes from all different sports, including runners, have discovered the impact of resistance training on their performance. Regardless of whether you run recreationally to maintain health and wellness, to manage your weight, to compete in local marathons, or to win an ultramarathon, you will benefit from adding resistance-training sessions to your weekly training plan. This is particularly true if training sessions are created with a specific purpose in mind and the plan reflects basic training principles.

The advantages gained by one person may be different from the benefit achieved by another. For example, one runner may improve biomechanics after initiating a resistance-training program while another may lose excess body fat. In the end, both improve running performance; each simply takes a different path to get there. Furthermore, the approach taken by each runner should be based on individual needs, interests, desires, and genetics.

Before any runner is willing to add another workout into a training plan, she/he must understand the potential benefits to be gained. This is not an exhaustive list of resistance-training benefits; instead it targets the fundamental benefits that most runners can expect to experience.

Improve running economy. Just as many people wish to have a car that is more economical, runners should strive to develop a movement pattern and cardiorespiratory system that is more economical. Often, runners hear about improving their fitness or their VO_2 max (maximum volume of oxygen consumed by the muscles during exercises) as a benefit of running. This variable is certainly an important indicator of cardiorespiratory fitness and mortality; those with better fitness live longer. However, running economy is a better predictor of running performance than VO_2 max. An improvement in running economy is seen when an individual runs faster at the same given level of oxygen consumption (or exertion).

Several explanations exist to explain how resistance training improves running economy. These include an improvement in biomechanics, muscle coordination (muscles that work well together), and recruitment of muscle fibers. By increasing muscular strength and coordination, a reduction in relative intensity occurs, which simply means you run faster with less effort! Research conducted on both recreational and highly trained runners has shown resistance training improves running economy by 3–10 percent. This translates into approximately a one to three-minute improvement for someone who runs a thirty-minute 5K. Individuals with less training will most likely see the greatest improvements.

Maintain or improve musculoskeletal fitness. In contrast to popular belief, cardiorespiratory (or aerobic) fitness is not the only type of fitness worth achieving. Healthy muscles, tendons, ligaments, connective tissue, and bones are just as critical to performance and wellness. In addition, a lack of musculoskeletal fitness will more often cause someone to take time off from running than a lack of cardiorespiratory fitness.

Muscle is an important part of the body's engine that burns fuel (calories) during rest and exercise. It is critical tissue to maintain (prevent loss) as well as to increase. The amount of muscle mass an individual has significantly impacts resting metabolism, which will ultimately influence energy balance and weight management. Unfortunately, as we age, the trend is to lose muscle mass and bone mass. Incorporating regular resistance training into your schedule will prevent this loss. Female runners in particular are at increased risk of stress fractures due to a combination of inadequate recovery time between training sessions, restriction of calories, poor bone health, and irregular menstrual cycles. Resistance training is an excellent way to improve bone health and minimize your risk by exposing the skeleton to weight-bearing loads that ultimately improve both bone and muscular strength.

Prevent or correct muscular imbalances. If running came in a bottle, many positive side effects would be listed on the label. Unfortunately, a few negative side effects can accompany the positive. The difference between other items found in a bottle and running (if it came packaged that way!) is that you can prevent the potential negative side effects of running.

Running is a repetitive movement pattern that takes place

primarily in one direction. This repetitive movement of certain muscle groups can actually lead to muscular imbalances and weaknesses in some individuals who spend a lot of time performing only this activity. The outcome is often characterized as one muscle group in a chronic shortened state while the opposing muscle group is in a chronic lengthened state. Furthermore, if someone has a postural deviation, running can further exacerbate the problem, possibly exhibiting itself in different areas of the body. For example, a runner with weak abdominal muscles (e.g., rectus abdominis) and tight hip flexor muscles (e.g., iliopsoas) may have an excessive forward tilt in the pelvis leading to compromised hamstring function.

Because running is primarily a movement that occurs in one direction, it is possible to forget about performing lateral (side to side) or rotational movement, which can lead to weak movement patterns in these directions. Many lateral muscles, particularly surrounding the hip, provide stability during running. Allowing these muscles to become weak will lead to a loss in power and speed during running and possibly an overuse injury like iliotibial (IT) band syndrome. A properly designed resistance-training program can prevent problems from occurring and correct weaknesses that may exist or develop.

Getting Started

At this point, you should be convinced that resistance training is good for running. The next step is to identify the basic principles behind designing a resistance-training program. Resistance training can be defined as any movement that requires the body's musculature to move (or attempt to) against an opposing force (resistance). The opposing force can be body weight, resistance tubing, weighted vest, medicine ball, plated weight stack, dumbbells, barbells, kettlebells, and the list goes on. Based on this definition, resistance training can take on a variety of training formats and be performed in many different places. This is beneficial for individuals trying to fit a resistance-training workout into their busy day. Let's consider three fundamental training principles important in designing a resistance-training program to enhance running performance.

1. **Individuality.** Each person experiences an individual response to a resistance-training stimulus or workout. This response will be dependent on the individual's age, fitness level, genetics, gender, and mental state. A program must be customized to the individual to encourage adherence and physiological adaptation.

2. **Specificity.** Physiological and metabolic responses (adaptations) are specific to muscle group, range of motion, and speed of muscle contraction performed. This principle is important on several levels. First, when selecting resistance-training exercises, it is important to choose movement patterns that are specific to running. This is done by selecting exercises that target muscles used within the range of motion, at the speed we want the muscles to contract, and functional to running movement. You do not lean against a wall while you run (at least not intentionally!), therefore, it is not useful to lean against a wall to perform a squat exercise. This is

not to say that cross-training activities are not important. But, when designing a resistance-training program, choose exercises that are similar to running movements. Furthermore, if you want to run faster, the goal is to recruit muscle fibers quickly in a coordinated pattern to create better muscular strength and power. This does not occur by performing repetitions at a very slow speed. Instead, perform repetitions at a speed that mimics running speed.

3. **Progressive overload.** The musculoskeletal system must be taxed with a greater force than it is accustomed to if it is to improve. Once the system adapts, it must be taxed again for continued improvement. Rest in between resistance-training sessions is critical for adaptation to occur. This principle is represented well with a staircase: step up by taxing the system (overload), rest to adapt (day off), then step up again to progress. You can tax the system by performing more repetitions, increasing the resistance, adding another set, decreasing the rest time between sets or exercises, incorporating different exercises, or increasing the frequency of resistance-training sessions. It is best to manipulate one of these variables at a time, not all at the same time! The goal is to challenge the neuromuscular system and keep it guessing but also to challenge your mental state to prevent boredom and disinterest.

If you still feel unsure of designing your own program, look for a fitness professional who is qualified to design a safe and effective resistance-training program, has experience working with runners, and is a runner.

Once you feel ready to begin a resistance-training program, you may ask yourself, *When do I have time to add in another training session or lengthen a current session to fit in resistance training?* Maybe you don't have to! For many runners, it is tough to give up a run for another activity. However, there is solid evidence that exchanging a run session with a resistance-training session improves performance more than maintaining a training plan that does not incorporate resistance training. Even though it may sound counterintuitive to run less but run better, it is worth a try! As you begin your next training plan, consider exchanging one run for one resistance-training session per week for four consecutive weeks. Ask yourself, *Did my performance deteriorate without that run? Did my performance benefit with that resistance-training session?*

Now, it is time to set a resistance-training goal. Keep it simple. *I will incorporate two resistance-training sessions per week for the next four weeks.* Create accountability for yourself by writing down your goal in your training log or discussing your goal with a friend or training partner. One of the keys to achieving your goal is checking in with yourself. After each week, reflect on your training to identify whether you met your goal for the week. If you did, continue working toward your goal the next week. If you did not, figure out why and attempt to avoid the same roadblocks the following week. Be patient with yourself as you begin a resistance-training program, but also remain persistent and consistent to achieve the benefits.

Whatever your running level, resistance training can help boost your cardio and muscular fitness. By incorporating resistance exercises into your weekly training schedule, you'll run stronger and better.

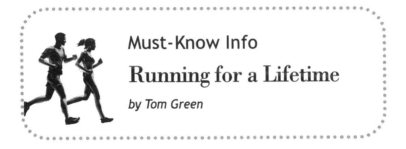

Must-Know Info

Running for a Lifetime

by Tom Green

Wraphen we are at the height of our running careers, we often take for granted our ability to continue running through the ages. Yet there's no Fountain of Youth to drink from to preserve our peak fitness. And there's no crystal ball to foresee what might sideline our running lives. Rather than count on luck or good fortune, there are a number of ways we can proactively extend our running success, enjoyment, and longevity through the years.

1. **Rotate your running shoes.** Owning more than one pair of running shoes and rotating them can provide more cushion to your runs. While it doesn't necessarily extend the life of the soles of your shoes, rotating can allow the cushion material to more fully recover than if your feet are pounding and compressing them day after day. Your joints will thank you.

2. **Use technical insoles in your shoes.** The factory insoles in your new shoes offer limited cushioning. Designed to fit the design of the shoe and your foot, factory insoles exist largely

to cover the rough manufacturing finish and stitching in the shoe. Today's new lightweight, high-impact absorbing insoles offer exponentially more cushion than the factory insoles and can increase comfort to your runs and extend the life of your shoes. Reputable brands include Sof Sole, Sorbothane, Spenco, and SuperFeet. The right insole can reduce the strain and inflammation on your muscles and add more miles to your running life.

3. **Maintain your stride.** No runner aspires to shuffle down the road, wobbling and with a running stride shorter than most walkers. Yet we've all seen them. Our running stride, the length between our extended lead foot and trailing foot, is often seen as the single-most important factor of maintaining strong running performance. As we age, our stride length decreases by as much as 10 percent per decade, resulting not only in slower running performances but also requiring more effort to transport our weight over our center of gravity. By losing stride length, we lose the momentum that propels our body forward, essentially "micro-braking" a little with each step and requiring more energy, cardio effort, and demand on our muscles to keep moving forward. The factor at play is weak muscles operating our joints, resulting in diminishing range of motion in our feet, hips, and knees. A simple method to restore this range of motion is through plyometrics, technique drills that build strength by exaggerating movement, such as in bounding and leaping. Another method is by running strides, quick, but short acceleration/deceleration runs of 80 to 100 meters. Finally, running

hills, both up and down, while paying close attention to good form and leg extension, can help us improve our stride length and efficiency.

4. **Get the help of sports medicine professionals.** Experienced physical therapists and athletic trainers are worth their weight in race medals. While you never want to ignore your family doc, sports medicine, physical therapy, and training professionals can work with you to keep running while addressing an injury or problem. The biggest payoff is that most of these professionals will not just treat your problem, but diagnose the cause to help prevent your problems from recurring. This is a far better solution than just laying off running.

5. **Leverage your strength.** To get the most out of your running, incorporate strength training, including for your core, into your routine. Runners often believe they are strong because they have endurance. Running long simply means you can repeat a motion over and over, mile after mile. That's confusing stamina with strength. The truth is many runners have strength deficiency and muscle imbalance in their legs, back, and hips, causing many of the injuries that set them back. Strength training is particularly important as runners age and we lose muscle mass. Twenty to thirty minutes of strength training several times per week will produce rapid, noticeable results and magnify your ability to run farther, faster, and longer for years.

6. **Regular massage for muscles.** There's nothing heroic in constantly having tight, strained muscles that are always on

the brink of tearing or breaking down. Muscles need to recover and return to their relaxed state to perform on demand. While only elite runners can afford and have access to regular, daily massage, ordinary runners can reap much of the same benefits by learning self-massage or using devices like The Stick. Found in most running stores, at large race expos, and online, The Stick is just one of several tools designed like a rolling pin to knead the muscles, loosening and energizing them by increasing blood flow to the tissue and reducing inflammation. Used regularly, self-massage or devices like The Stick can keep legs fresh day after day and throughout the years.

7. **Use progressive runs.** When you can't, shouldn't, or prefer not to run gritty intervals, repeats, and tempo workouts, progressive runs are an alternative to help you maintain and even increase speed. Progressive runs are simply the practice of picking up the pace for the later part of an easy, putting-in-the-miles run. With no precise formula, progressive runs involve gradually increasing pace over the last 10 to 25 percent of your run. These runs are optimal for nearly every runner because they produce a cardio benefit, generate more rapid leg turnover, and conclude with a strong, exhilarating finish when the muscles and systems are warmed up and not as likely to lead to injury.

8. **Use an experienced coach.** You know the adage, "We don't know what we don't know," so sometimes it takes an objective person to help us understand principles and practices that work consistently and predictably for runners. A skilled

and experienced running coach can identify when and how to train to peak and how to get the most benefit from recovery, including off-season running. A coach's wisdom can also anticipate problems you might experience and help address them before you are sidelined or slowed down. Certified coaches can be found at the Road Runner Clubs of America (http://www.rrca.org), and by inquiring at your local running store.

9. **Race less often but still with stretch goals.** What is more exciting than a full slate of races to run weekend after weekend? As we age, that kind of schedule becomes a distant memory. But we can still extend our years of racing and also enjoy success by targeting key races for which we prepare and peak. Our preferred races can become great annual traditions and allow us to focus and prepare as well as when we were younger and our race card was full every weekend.

Most runners don't see an end to their running careers—and for good reason. By understanding some of the components of extending the running life—and acting on them—most runners can enjoy the fitness, accomplishments, and euphoria of running for a lifetime.

The Writers

Becky Green Aaronson is a freelance writer living in Santa Barbara, California. Her work has appeared in *Runner's World* and several other publications. She has completed seven marathons and her running has taken her everywhere from Paris to Rome to Mount Everest Base Camp. When she's not chasing after adventures, she's working on two books.

Brian Aldrich was 300 pounds in 2005 when he started running. He ran his first marathon on the Great Wall of China in 2009 when he weighed 280 pounds. Brian's inspiration comes from his father, who is a runner, and also his mother, whose weight-loss journey also inspires many.

Dana Barclay, a dedicated runner, splits her time between Michigan and the Caribbean, mixing her running routine with scuba diving and yoga. She has a master's degree in agronomy and lives in semiretirement after spending some twenty-odd years in agriculture. Other interests include animal husbandry and botany. You can contact Dana at danabarclay@hotmail.com.

Carol M. Benthal-Bingley lives in Rockford, Illinois, with her husband and three daughters. She is an artist, mother, runner, and the founder of Annie's Locker (http://www.annieslocker.org), a non-profit that collects and distributes new and used fitness gear to people in need. She is delighted that Annie's Locker and "Running for Two" has blossomed into a ministry that serves others. Several years ago, God gave her these words: "Create. Inspire." That's what she strives to do. Write to Carol at carol@b2design.com.

Bridgette L. Collins is president and founder of MAC Fitness, a fitness consulting firm in Grand Prairie, Texas. She is a recognized fitness coach, motivational speaker, and writer who loves to participate in half and full marathons. She is the author of *Destined to Live Healthier* and *Imagine Living Healthier*, two books that have empowered many through the collection of fictional stories that tell of real life challenges with weight, health, work, marriage, and lack of self-love. You may contact Bridgette by e-mail at Bridgette@bridgettecollins.com or www.BridgetteCollins.com.

Chryselle D'Silva Dias is a freelance writer and blogger based in Goa, India, whose work has appeared in national and international publications. She likes writing about travel, green issues, design, literacy, books, and lifestyles, but can write about almost anything. Visit her at http://www.chryselle.net.

Lisa Finch lives in Forest, Ontario, Canada, with her wonderful husband Chris and their three beautiful children, Hailey, Matthew, and Ben. This is Lisa's fifth story published in an anthology. For more information, please visit her at www.finchtales. webs.com.

Heather Gannoe is an avid runner and proud mommy to two toddler boys. She is currently training for her first season of triathlon competitions while fundraising for Team Fight. Heather is also pursuing her degree in exercise and sports science from Coastal Carolina University, with the hope to share her love for running and fitness with others. You can follow her adventures at her website, www.runfaster mommy.com.

Sean Geary lives and works in Ann Arbor, Michigan. When he is not eating things he probably shouldn't eat from the hands of strangers, he can be found around Ann Arbor or in Northern Michigan on a bicycle or running with his son Kellan (The Dude) and their three dogs.

Miriam Hill is the coauthor of *Fabulous Florida* and a frequent contributor to Chicken Soup for the Soul books. She's been published in *Christian Science Monitor*, *Grit*, *St. Petersburg Times*, *Sacramento Bee*, and Poynter Online. Miriam's manuscript received an honorable mention for inspirational writing in a *Writer's Digest* writing competition.

Joanne Hirase-Stacey is a running writer who lives in southeast Idaho. She enjoys writing fiction, nonfiction, poetry, and devotionals, and has published several pieces of work. She also quilts and paints, and she just took up karate. She doesn't believe in sitting on the sidelines of life, so she's living life her way.

Harry Jacobs is a self-professed computer geek who enjoys many activities including running, reading, acting, and online computer role-playing games. Harry is lucky, as his wife supports many of his eccentric behaviors.

Rachel E. Jones lives a seminomadic lifestyle in the Horn of Africa with her husband and three children. Her articles have appeared in *Running Times*, the Chicken Soup for the Soul series, and parenting magazines. Write to Rachel at djibouti@ reiinc.org.

Kim Dent Karrick is a graduate from Louisiana State University, where she was the first female sports editor for LSU's newspaper, *The Daily Reveille*. She was inspired by her father's love of all sports to participate in sports in some form . . . her lack of athletic prowess led her to choose writing about them. She is a long-time resident of Covington, Louisiana, where she lives with her husband of nineteen years, Bobby. They love biking and swimming together, but she leaves the running to him!

Amanda Krieger is a freelance writer living in Richmond, Virginia. She is a recent graduate of Virginia Tech and enjoys running, hiking, mountain biking, and rock climbing.

Katherine Locke lives in the United Kingdom with her family. She was diagnosed with breast cancer in 2007 and took up running after the completion of her treatment to get fit as quickly as possible. She is still running at least three times a week and has come a long way since she wrote this piece!

Frank McKinney, known as the Daredevil Real Estate Artist, is a five-time international bestselling author, philanthropist, risk-taker, and visionary who sees opportunities and creates markets where none existed before. He has been the subject of numerous international television, radio, and print features, including ABC's *20/20*, *USA Today*, the *Oprah Winfrey Show*, CBS' *The Early Show*, CNN, Discovery Channel, Travel Channel, HGTV, CBN TV, NPR, *Wall Street Journal*, *New York Times*, *Fortune*, *Barrons*, and *Town and Country*. In 1998, Frank and his wife, Nilsa, founded Caring House Project Foundation, a nonprofit (501c3) organization that provides housing and a self-sustaining existence for homeless families in South America, the Caribbean, Africa, Indonesia, and the United States. Learn more at www. Frank-McKinney.com.

Mary Monaghan is a writer and professional speaker. She is the author of *Remember Me?* and *Who Do You Belong To?* She is also a contributor to *Life Choices—Navigating Difficult Paths*. Contact Mary at www.marymonaghan.com or marymonaghan @telkomsa.net, or by writing to: P. O. Box 163, Melkbosstrand, 7437, South Africa.

Dani Nichols is a freelance writer who loves her husband, good coffee, country music, free museums, and long road trips. She writes nearly every day at www. wranglerdani.com, teaches therapeutic horseback riding, and relearns how to be a runner.

Perry P. Perkins, novelist, blogger, and award-winning travel writer, is a stay-at-home dad who lives with his wife, Victoria, and their one-year-old daughter, Grace, in the Pacific Northwest. His novels include *Just Past Oysterville*, *Shoalwater Voices*, and *The Light at the End of the Tunnel*. Perry has written for numerous magazines and anthologies. His inspirational stories have been included in eleven Chicken Soup anthologies as well. Examples of his published work can be found online at www.perryperkinsbooks.com and on his blog: www.ricecereal.wordpress.com

Jeff Pickett is a father of six and an advocate for health. His passions for running, fitness, and working out are fueled by his desire to spend more time with his family and be an example for them. When Jeff isn't working as a nonprofit marketer, he enjoys eating well, playing hard, and laughing often. His blog on running, working out, and eating healthy can be found at http://lifeisntover.wordpress.com.

Connie K. Pombo is a contributing author to numerous compilations and author of *Trading Ashes for Roses* and *Moms of Sons Devotions to Go*. She is a freelance writer and mentoring specialist who runs to keep up with her two sons. You can reach her at http://www.conniepombo.com.

Jonathon Prince is a social *athlivist* (athlete-activist) who continues to promote change worldwide, one country at a time. Through his now seasoned fund-raiser titled "Hope or Die," Jonathon spreads the spirit of hope and change while raising monetary donations for individuals in distress. While changing the biased thinking that only the fortunate can aid in humanitarian works, Jonathon confirms that the courage to act in faith not only creates avenues to help others, but also allows one to satisfy one's personal obligation to live life selflessly and abundantly. Learn more at www.hopeordie.com and www.wechoosehope.com

Marcia Puryear has been a runner for more than twenty-five years, both competitively and just for fun and friendship. She has run eight marathons, winning three in her age groups. Her most recent win, at age sixty-four, was the San Francisco Marathon in 2006. She retired from twenty-five years of teaching last June, and looks forward to many more years of involvement with her running life to include helping others follow their own dreams and goals with her coaching business, Coachlink. She lives in Concord, Massachusetts, with her husband, and has two grown children and a new first granddaughter. You can e-mail Marcia at coachat@comcast.net.

Joseph F. Rottino is a retired New York City high school English teacher, track and field, and soccer coach. Joe has stumbled his way through some fifty marathons and ultramarathons, including the New York City, Marine Corps, New Orleans Mardi Gras, Vegas Marathon, and the Great Philadelphia to Atlantic City 100K Road Race. In the course of his meanderings, he has logged some 40,000 miles on various American roads and tracks.

Marcia Rudoff is a newspaper columnist, memoir-writing instructor, and freelance writer in Bainbridge Island, Washington. She is the author of *We Have Stories: A Handbook for Writing Your Memoirs*. In spite of her reluctant debut as a runner at the age of sixty, she celebrated turning sixty-five by competing in her first marathon.

Mike Rush is a public school teacher, father, husband, and writer.

Lana Matthews Sain is a mother of two boys, a full-time computer programmer, and an avid marathon runner and triathlete. She completed Ironman Florida in 2008. She enjoys writing about her experiences as a mom/runner/triathlete at her blog called "The Fire Inside": http://lanasmarathonjourney.blogspot.com.

Felicia Schneiderhan grew up on the Mississippi River, the daughter of a nun who was caught by a fisherman. She currently lives in northern Minnesota with her husband, Mark. Her short stories, essays, and articles have appeared in all kinds of journals and magazines.

Ericka Umbarger was diagnosed with juvenile rheumatoid arthritis in 1993 at the age of thirteen. She was very active before her diagnosis and always dreamed about running a marathon one day. She has achieved that, and more.

Samantha Ducloux Waltz, an award-winning freelance writer in Portland, Oregon, currently has more than forty essays in the Ultimate series, the Chicken Soup for the Soul series, A Cup of Comfort series, and numerous other anthologies. She has also written fiction and nonfiction under the name Samellyn Wood. Learn more at www.pathsofthought.com.

Christy Whiteman is a thirty-six–year-old wife and mother with a seven-year-old boy and a four-year-old girl. She has a full-time career outside of the home and stays active and busy in her community. She is also an avid runner and has completed one marathon, a few half-marathons, and several other races. She absolutely loves her life!

Larry Williams lives in Stoney Creek, Ontario, Canada, with his lovely wife, Kathleen, and their wonderful children, Nicole and Tyler. With the support and encouragement of his family, Larry has been running for six years. Since the writing of this story, he has completed a few more races. The Boston Marathon is still on his "to-do" list.

Megan Williams is a marathoner and Ironman triathlete who lives in Philadelphia with her husband, twenty-month-old twins, and four cats. She teaches at Temple University, and her work has been published in *Contemporary Literature*, *Modern Drama*, *Alligator Juniper*, and *Aethlon: The Journal of Sport Literature*.

Pat Williams is the senior vice president of the Orlando Magic, and has been a marathon runner in fifty-five races.

Christopher Wink is the media director at Back on My Feet and a resident of Philadelphia's Fishtown neighborhood. Back on My Feet is a nonprofit organization that promotes the self-sufficiency of homeless populations by engaging them in running as a means to build confidence, strength, and self-esteem. Participating members can earn eligibility in education, housing, job training, and job placement programs. Based in Philadelphia, the organization has chapters in Washington D.C., Boston, Baltimore, and elsewhere. For more information, visit www.backonmyfeet.org.

Tonya Woodworth is the editorial assistant for HCI Books. As a former marine, Tonya served in both Operation Enduring Freedom and Operation Iraqi Freedom, which fueled her immense passion for travel. She most recently visited Brazil, where she was able to fulfill her desire to better understand the country, its language, and its culture. Visit her at www.TonyaWoodworth.com for an in-depth view of her travels.

The Photographers

Brian Aldrich was 300 pounds when he started running in 2005. He ran his first marathon in 2009 on the Great Wall of China; he weighed 280 pounds. Brian's inspiration comes from his father who is a runner, and also from his mother, whose weight loss journey also inspires many.

Lee Brown is affiliated with the Halesowen Athletics and Cycling Club (www.halesowen-athleticclub.co.uk/). Lee has two sons who run for the club, representing the club, their district, county, and country . . . England. Lee began taking photos of his sons and their teammates during events, and got into running in order to run the courses for better shots. He enjoys how; in this multimedia world we live in, still photography is as popular as ever, particularly with the kids. The shot published here features athletes (U15 Boys) in their district colors, racing for places in the county team of Worcestershire.

Dave Getzschman is a San Francisco-based photographer who provides fresh, compelling imagery for clients spanning the editorial, corporate, and commercial markets. To each shoot, Getzschman brings empathy for his subjects, humor appropriate for the occasion, and a sense of joy for the creative process. To see his latest work, visit http://pa.photoshelter.com/user/davegetzschman.

Paula Jansen's goal as a commercial photographer is to illustrate her client's vision in the most artistic and creative way possible. Paula uses a mixture of natural and strobe lights to render objects in a lifelike manner. She began her career working on children's books and enjoys collaborating on projects with art directors and editors. Her photography is featured in *Sharing the Table at Garland's Lodge*, which was a 2006 finalist for the IACP Cookbook Award. Please visit Paula's website, www.paulajansen.com, to enjoy more of her photography and her visual blog.

Ron Leonhardt has had an interest in photography for the past thirty-five years. With several thousand photographs of runners, bikers, and swimmers to choose from, Ron's challenge is finding that special photo for his local running club's newsletter that puts a smile on readers' faces. With so much to learn about composition, lighting, f-stops, and shutter speeds, Ron is grateful that he has an enthusiastic group of athletes eager to serve as his training subjects at a moment's notice.

Don Lundell is a photographer and ultra runner, and co-owner of ZombieRunner, a store for runners in Palo Alto, California. You can see more of his photographic work at www.zombierunner.com.

Bud Morton is a freelance photographer from the southeast Massachusetts area. Bud enjoys photographing running events for his running club, the Colonial Road Runners. He also photographs professional horse-racing events including some Triple Crown races and the Breeders' Cup. View Bud's work at www.budmorton-photography.com

Brad Presner is an avid triathlete, having completed four marathons and more than twenty triathlons from sprint to Ironman distances. When not working as a manager of a nonprofit organization or training, Brad is an avid hobbyist photographer who is currently focused on taking as many pictures of his newborn son as he can.

Denis Prézat is an amateur photographer living in Paris, France. He has been interested in photography since he was a teenager and even managed to get through his military service wielding a camera. Denis's favorite topics to snap are sporting events and street art.

Michael Scott is a freelance photographer whose work regularly appears in national and regional track and field/running publications. He chairs the USATF Cross Country Council (since 2003) and is an academic advisor for student athletes at the University of Rhode Island. The photo published here was taken at the 2009 IAAF Cross Country Championships in Amman, Jordan. His track and field photos may be viewed at http://miscottrunningphoto.shutterfly.com.

The Must-Know Experts

Shawn H. Dolan, Ph.D., R.D., CSSD, is an assistant professor of kinesiology at California State University, Long Beach, and a sports dietitian. Her areas of teaching expertise include sport and wellness nutrition, resistance training program design, and personal training. Shawn's research focuses on the role nutrition and exercise play in performance with an emphasis on endurance athletes and fitness professionals. Shawn is an avid runner and triathlete. Her favorite distances to compete in include half marathon and 70.3 Half Ironman.

Brian Dorfman is unsurpassed in his ability to prevent, diagnose, and treat sports related injuries. For over twenty-five years, world-class athletes have relied on Brian's techniques to keep them performing at their peak. For more information, to schedule an appointment, or to purchase the Flexibility Training DVD, visit www.briandorfman.com.

Lisa Dorfman, M.S., R.D., CSSD, LMHC, has been the sports nutritionist for the University of Miami athletic department, an adjunct professor in the exercise and sport sciences, and is the director of sports nutrition and performance. She is also a consultant to U.S. Sailing and professional athletes worldwide. Lisa is a former pro triathlete and a competitor in more than thirty marathons (PR 2:52:32), Ironman USA, and the 2004 Long Distance Duathlon World Championships for Team USA. Lisa has been featured on *Dateline*, *20/20*, CNN, ESPN, Fox, MSNBC, *Designing Spaces*, E!, and local and international news. Her writing appears in dozens of publications monthly, including *SoBeFit* magazine where she is Nutrition Editor. Lisa's books, *The Reunion Diet* (www.TheReunionDiet.com), *The Tropical Diet*, and *The Vegetarian Sports Nutrition Guide* and programs are available worldwide and at her website: www.foodfitness.com.

Janet Hamilton, M.A., RCEP, CSCS, ACSM Registered Clinical Exercise Physiologist, has thirty years of experience working with athletes of all ages and abilities, is an RRCA-certified distance running coach, and serves as an instructor for the RRCA Coaching Certification program. She earned her master's degree in exercise physiology in 1987, and is a Registered Clinical Exercise Physiologist (RCEP) through the American College of Sports Medicine. She has been a Certified Strength and Conditioning Specialist (CSCS) through the National Strength and

Conditioning Association since 1993, and has been a member of the American Physical Therapy Association since 1978. She has been coaching runners through her business Running Strong for sixteen years. She is the author of the book *Running Strong & Injury-Free*, currently in its third printing. Visit Janet at www.runningstrong.com.

Jason R. Karp, Ph.D., is a nationally-recognized speaker, writer, and exercise physiologist who coaches recreational runners to Olympic hopefuls through his company, RunCoachJason.com. He holds a Ph.D. in exercise physiology and is director and coach of REVO2LT Running Team. He writes for numerous international running, coaching, and fitness magazines and scientific journals, and is a frequent presenter at running and fitness conferences. He is also the author of *101 Developmental Concepts and Workouts for Cross Country Runners*. Subscribe to his free e-mail newsletter at www.runcoachjason.com/newsletter.

Claire Kowalchik is the author of the bestselling book, *The Complete Book of Running for Women*. Claire is a former managing editor of *Runner's World* magazine. She has run eight marathons, including Boston, and countless races from the mile to the half-marathon. She lives in Emmaus, Pennsylvania, with her two sons, Michael and Benjamin, who occasionally join her for a run.

Clint Verran is an elite runner, expert coach, and sports medicine professional. He holds a master's degree in physical therapy (MPT) and operates Clint Verran Sports Medicine, a company dedicated to the health and wellness of athletes of all ages and abilities. A member of the *Runner's World* advisory board and a frequent contributor to *Runner's World* magazine, Clint has raced competitively around the globe. His personal best (PB) is a 13:51 5K, and some of his impressive finishes include seventeenth in the 2000 IAAF World Half Marathon Championships; twenty-second in the 2005 IAFF World Championship Marathon; and fifth in the 2004 U.S. Olympic Trials Men's Marathon. He placed tenth in the 2006 Boston Marathon with a time of 2:14:12. Clint provides coaching services and is highly regarded for helping runners achieve their goals. Learn more about Clint at www.runguru.com

Copyright Credits

Index

About the Authors

Tom Green has been an ordinary runner for thirty-six years. He is the cocreator of Runners' Lounge, an online community founded in 2007 for runners to meet others, to build running communities, and to talk about what consistently, predictably works for runners. Tom runs consistently and quietly in his home community of Des Moines, Iowa, and races occasionally, but always makes time for his favorite race, the Chicago Marathon. He and his wife, Mary, a nonrunner, have three children, Laura, Daniel, and Elizabeth, who were all runners during school. Tom works in the human resources profession, focusing on leadership development and performance consulting in Des Moines, Iowa. When not working or running, Tom enjoys gardening and writing. For more information, contact Tom at: tom@runnerslounge.com.

Amy Hunold-VanGundy is possibly the world's slowest runner but still enjoys the time she gets to spend on the roads and trails in her hometown. Amy tries to fit her running around work, kids, and life, and sometimes is successful. She cocreated Runners' Lounge as a way to make it easier for runners to connect to others and share their challenges and victories. It was in this creation that she found so many other runners in the world who share her passion for running but may not share the speed of others. She also found that all runners have a story and these stories continue to feed her passion for all things running. Amy works in human resources and business consulting in Des Moines, Iowa. She and her husband, Jim, have two children, Tucker and Sophie. When she's not working or running, Amy enjoys reading. She can be contacted at: amy@runnerslounge.com.

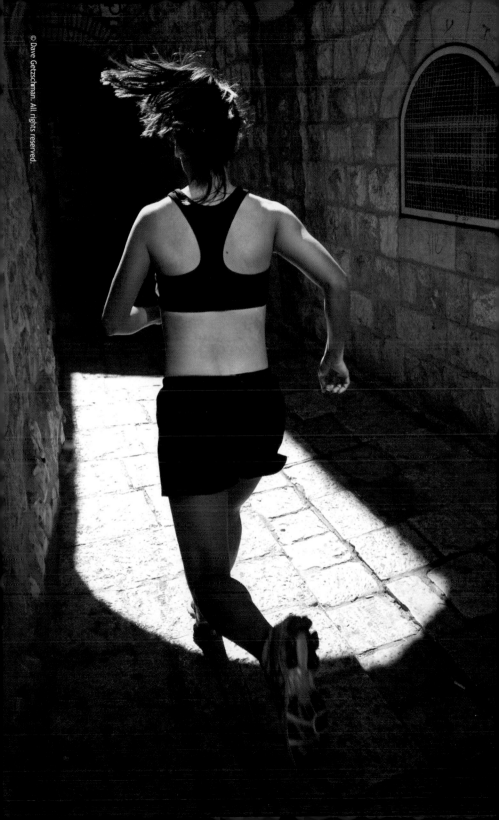

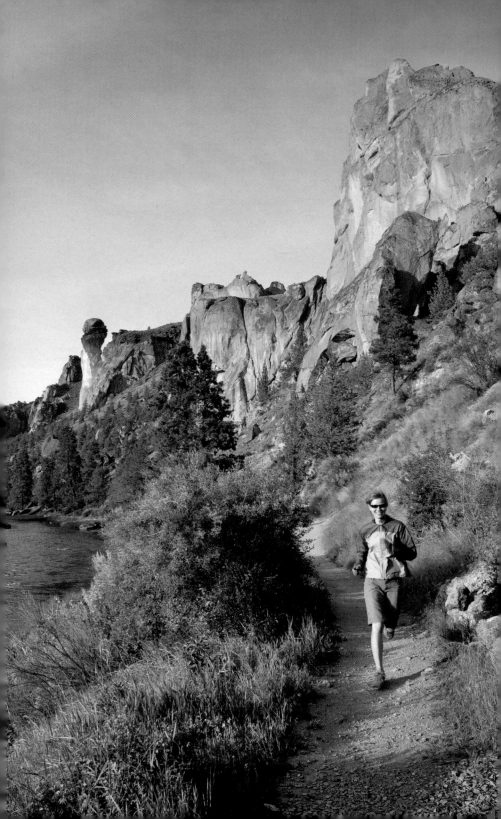

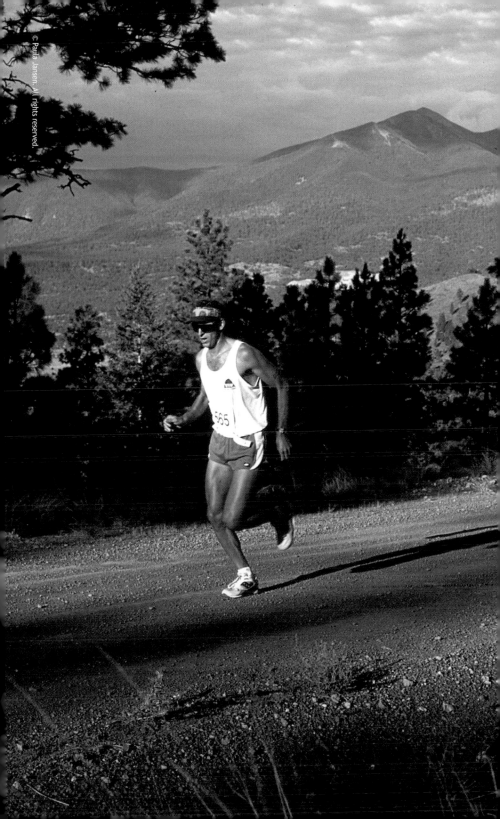

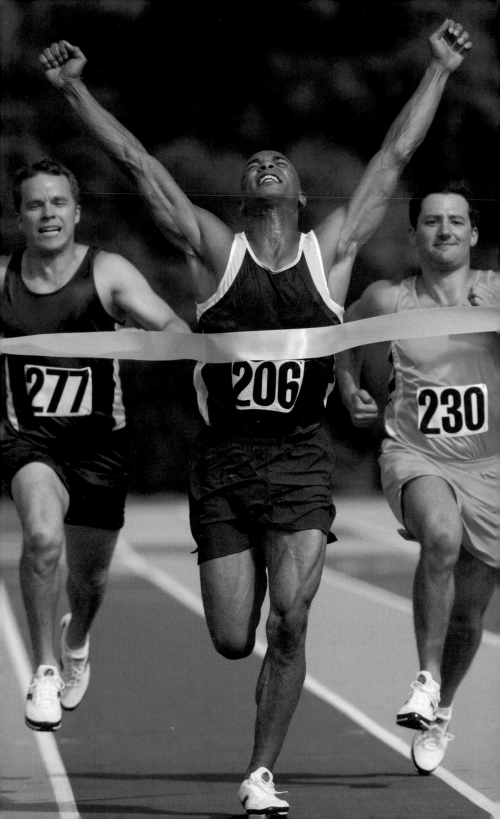